Every Woman's Guide to

DIABETES

D1059231

This book is meant to educate, but it should not be used as a substitute for personal medical advice. Readers should consult their physicians for specific information concerning their individual medical conditions. The authors have done their best to ensure that the information presented here is accurate up to the time of publication. However, as research and development are ongoing, it is possible that new findings may supersede some of the data presented here.

Many of the designations used by manufacturers and sellers to distinguish their products are claimed as trademarks. Where those designations appear in this book and Harvard University Press was aware of a trademark claim, then the designations have been printed in initial capital letters (for example, Tylenol).

Every Woman's Guide to
DIABETES

What You Need to Know to Lower Your Risk and Beat the Odds

STEPHANIE A. EISENSTAT, M.D.

DAVID M. NATHAN, M.D., Consulting Editor

ELLEN BARLOW

HARVARD UNIVERSITY PRESS
Cambridge, Massachusetts London, England

Drawings by Arleen Frasca

"Are You Living on the Edge? A Self-Diagnosis Checklist" is
reprinted on pages 170–171, with permission, from Joslin Diabetes
Center's website, www.joslin.org. Copyright © 2006 by Joslin
Diabetes Center, Inc.

First Harvard University Press paperback edition, 2008.

Library of Congress Cataloging-in-Publication Data

Eisenstat, Stephanie A.
    Every woman's guide to diabetes : what you need to know to
      lower your risk and beat the odds / Stephanie A. Eisenstat,
      David M. Nathan (consulting editor), Ellen Barlow.
        p.   cm.
    Includes bibliographical references and index.
    ISBN 978-0-674-02304-8 (cloth : alk. paper)
    ISBN 978-0-674-02728-2 (pbk.)
    1. Diabetes in women—Popular works.   I. Title.

RC660.4.E37   2007
616.4'62—dc22   2006049463

To our families:

Russell, Benjamin, Samuel, and Joshua Eisenstat
Alex and Charlie Boyajian and Charles and Margaret Barlow

To the women in Dr. Nathan's life:

Rhoda and Ellen

To the patients with diabetes, and colleagues, who have taught Drs. Eisenstat
and Nathan over the years

Contents

Preface by Stephanie A. Eisenstat ix
Preface by David M. Nathan xii

1 The New Epidemic 1

2 Diagnosis 18

3 Prevention 37

4 Medical Complications 74

5 Reproductive Health and Sexuality 112

6 Psychosocial Impact 150

7 Management of the Disease 178

8 Common Questions and Resources 225

APPENDIXES

1 Body Mass Index (BMI) Table 259

2 Carbohydrate Counts for Common Fruits,
Vegetables, Starches, and Dairy 262

3 Sample Grocery List for Healthful Eating 264

4 Choosing a Blood Glucose Meter 266

5 Mixing Different Kinds of Insulin 269

6 Disposing of Syringes 270

7 Insulin Pumps and Other Insulin Delivery Systems 271

8 Over-the-Counter Medications and Diabetes 273

9 Complementary (Alternative Medicine) Treatments 274

10 Your Diabetic Targets 276

Glossary of Terms 277
References 289
Acknowledgments 298
Index 299

Preface by Stephanie A. Eisenstat

When I was first told I had diabetes, I was in shock and so was my family. I was a new mother in my thirties, and no one in my family had diabetes. For months I had been experiencing weight loss, fatigue, increased urination at night, headaches, joint aches, and frequent yeast infections. Despite being a doctor and knowing better, I thought all these problems were due to my stressful life—raising my children, caring for ill family members, working full time, having a husband who traveled for business, and generally being the one who holds all the pieces together. I viewed myself as a strong, healthy person with relatively healthy living habits. I visited my doctor at most once a year for that annual pap and flu shot.

All that changed after diagnosis. In my case, I went right on insulin and battled with high and low blood sugars, a new eating schedule at home and work, and frightening information from specialists about all the potential complications of this disease. The first time I saw the eye doctor, despite his best intentions he proceeded to recite a litany of awful things that would happen to me, including blindness, if I didn't take this diagnosis seriously. And although I knew all this as a doctor, hearing it as a patient was different and, frankly, increased my denial of the disease. Over the ensuing months, with the help and understanding of my health care team, I came to realize that the signs and symptoms I had been experiencing all led to the same conclusion, confirmed by a simple blood test: I really did have diabetes. I had to come to terms with my illness before it got out of control and impacted my physical well being, emotional outlook, friends, family, co-workers—in short, my entire life.

Looking back, I consider myself lucky. I had symptoms that brought me to the doctor, whereas for many people diabetes is a silent killer. I live in Boston, a mecca of medical care, with superb doctors and health care teams, whereas many Americans are without health insurance and must bear the high cost of drugs and diabetes supplies themselves. I started on insulin and soon felt much better. Some people don't feel back to normal for some time.

I quickly realized, however, that diabetes can be emotionally wearing at best and downright oppressive and frightening at worst. All of a sudden (and for the rest of your life), you need medical care, and you have to learn how to navigate a complex medical care system. You also have to self-manage diabetes outside the doctor's office: monitoring glucose at home, watching what you eat, taking medication, understanding your symptoms and communicating with your health care team, exercising when you don't have an extra minute in your day, and maintaining a strong conviction that you will beat this disease and prevent all the complications associated with it.

Many of the patients with diabetes whom I care for in my own general medicine practice share my sentiment. They, too, are frustrated because on a day-to-day basis they find it difficult to meet diabetic targets: the $HgbA_{1C}$ under 7 percent, fasting blood sugars less than 100–120, normal cholesterol panel, ideal body weight, and so on. They sometimes feel lost and deflated. They don't get a chance to hear from those who are successfully managing their disease. They may not yet realize that even though everyone's situation is unique, they are not alone, that, with psychological support, diabetes education programs, and a good medical team, they can become active participants in their care rather than passive observers.

About two years ago I approached Dr. David Nathan, one of my colleagues, a superb clinician, researcher, and leading expert in the diabetes world, and asked if he and Ellen Barlow, a medical writer, would work with me on a book to help women better understand diabetes and its complex management issues. Together we created *Every Woman's Guide to Diabetes* to empower women to self-manage diabetes in partnership with their medical team, and to more readily translate "diabetes awareness" into action.

This book is the "what, why, and how to" of diabetes care for women. We cover the unique aspects of the disease for women, the nature of diabetes, its causes and potential consequences, the complexity of medical decision making and treatment, and the challenge of core lifestyle changes critical to successful prevention of complications. We also suggest strategies to decrease stress and feelings of isolation, and offer management techniques for home and work. We talk about the dreaded "diabetes diet" and explore how to make smart tradeoffs when choosing what to eat. We highlight the relationships between what you do during the course of a day, how you feel, and their impact on glucose control. We also let you know how to reduce your risk factors for heart disease, the number one killer of women with diabetes. And we provide tips for starting an exercise program and advice for making the most of your medical visits.

We hope this book helps you and your families avoid the pitfalls that I and others have encountered over the years.

This book is for any woman who has diabetes or may be at risk for diabetes, and any family member who wants to learn how to help make diabetes more manageable at home for their loved ones. It is meant to complement the information you receive from members of your medical care team, who know your situation best. More important, the aim of this book is to make those of you with diabetes realize that you can feel physically and emotionally better. By learning effective strategies, you can control this disease rather than feeling that the disease is controlling you.

Be healthy!

Stephanie A. Eisenstat, M.D.

Preface by David M. Nathan

When Stephanie Eisenstat first proposed a book on women and diabetes, I didn't understand the need for a separate guide focusing on women's issues specifically. After all, type 1 and type 2 diabetes affect women and men in similar proportions. The relationship between diabetes control and complications is much the same for both sexes, and there are few, if any, major differences in therapy for women and men. The most obvious difference between the sexes is the occurrence of a unique form of diabetes, gestational diabetes, in women. But as we discussed the variety of ways that diabetes affects women and, conversely, how being a woman affects the experience of the disease, I realized that there were numerous topics that deserved—in fact, demanded—special attention.

The most recent estimates are that 25–30 percent of all people born at the beginning of the twenty-first century will develop diabetes during their lifetime. One half of them will be women. This book aims to address diabetes issues that are relevant to all people, such as how to prevent or delay the development of type 2 diabetes, how to improve your chances of living a healthy life without complications, and how to incorporate diabetes care comfortably and safely into your everyday life. However, we focus in particular on topics that have special significance for women, such as diabetes during pregnancy, the effect of the menstrual cycle on diabetes control, and how diabetes, and perhaps prediabetes, may erase the protective effect of being a woman as it relates to heart disease. Since diabetes has a great impact on daily life, many of the insights and much of the advice we offer are tailored to women and their lifestyles. As similar as women's and men's lives have become in the workplace, there are still numerous differences between your day and those of a man that may affect your diabetes. We hope we have been sensitive to those differences and have provided a book that will help you manage your diabetes successfully.

I am mindful that most people who read this book, if only because of its title, will be women; however, it wouldn't hurt men to read it as well, for much of the information also applies to them. In addition, if you're a man and have a partner or other family member with diabetes, the descriptions we provide may help you understand a little better what your wife, daughter, or mother is experiencing and make you a more empathetic, supportive partner.

David M. Nathan, M.D.

1

The New Epidemic

Claire, age forty-two, is a working mother of three teenagers who also cares for her legally blind father. At 5'3" and 250 pounds, she has been trying to lose weight for years. An aunt, two uncles, and her father all have diabetes. Even so, she was shocked when a routine blood glucose test came back high at 300, indicating that she has diabetes. Panic set in, as she began to worry about how her family would cope should she be unable to work.

Perhaps you, too, have just been told you have diabetes or that you are at risk for it. If so, you are not alone. Nearly twenty-one million Americans are living with this same reality, and a little over half of them are women. Another forty-one million Americans have prediabetes and are at high risk for developing the disease.

You are one of the lucky ones. About one-third of women with diabetes don't even know they have it. You may not feel very lucky, but at least you are ahead of the game. You *know* you have to make some changes to stay healthy. We can show you how.

You don't have to be a superwoman to prevent diabetes or stay healthy with the disease. But from now on you *do* have to pay attention to your body and what it needs. Though uninvited, diabetes has brought change into your life. But it is within your power to make lemonade from this lemon—and it does not have to be unsweetened! What you learn and apply to your life will help you prevent the disease or problems associated with it. What's more, you can share your new knowledge with family members to help them live healthier lives, too.

This chapter contains statistics and information that shows you why physicians, researchers, public health experts, and government officials are so concerned about the dramatic rise in diabetes. After this chapter, we will concentrate more on you—the realities you face in living day to day with diabetes or its threat.

WHY A BOOK FOR WOMEN?

Women have a far greater risk of developing diabetes than breast cancer, typically the most feared disease among women. If current trends continue, one in three women born today can expect to develop diabetes at some point in her life.

In general, women are slightly more likely than men to develop diabetes. But among some ethnic groups, women are at a substantially increased risk for the disease. Hispanic women born since 2000, for example, have an estimated fifty-fifty chance of developing diabetes in their lifetime. African American, American Indian, and Asian American women, as well as those from the Pacific Rim, also have a higher-than-average risk of developing diabetes.

Women with diabetes or at risk for diabetes face some unique problems. Diabetes can negatively affect a woman's reproductive health and sexuality. It can also affect her children both before and after birth. Women with gestational diabetes, a form of the disease that develops during pregnancy, have a high risk of developing diabetes in the years following delivery.

The rising tide of diabetes

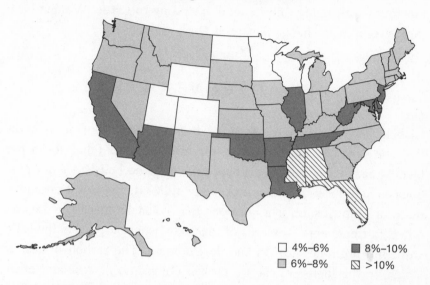

☐ 4%–6%	■ 8%–10%
☐ 6%–8%	◩ >10%

Percentage of Americans with diabetes, by state. (Data from the Centers for Disease Control and Prevention.)

Some of the medical problems related to having diabetes—such as heart disease—may also affect women more severely than men. After a heart attack, for example, women with diabetes are less likely to survive and more likely to have a poorer quality of life than men with diabetes. Diabetes appears to erase the protective effect of being a woman as it relates to heart disease.

Although 70 percent of women with diabetes have private, job-based health insurance, many women in high-risk groups do not have health insurance. Women in high-risk groups are also more likely than men to rely on government health insurance programs. Inadequate insurance coverage is a potential roadblock women face in managing their diabetes successfully.

Women are often the ones in a position to make healthful changes in the household, such as in the food cooked and served. Healthy eating habits are especially important given the alarming rise in type 2 diabetes in children under age nineteen. The increase may be attributed to the fact that children and teenagers are eating too much, especially fast foods with many calories, and exercising too little. Women have the power to help change this trend.

WHAT'S GONE AWRY

Diabetes mellitus is really a group of diseases. But in general, we know that someone has diabetes when the level of sugar (glucose) in her bloodstream is elevated. This happens when the body does not produce enough insulin, does not properly utilize the insulin it does produce, or both. Insulin is a hormone that normally helps glucose and other nutrients enter the cells of the body, where it powers the cells' work and promotes growth and development. The carbohydrates, or starch, in the foods we eat are broken down into glucose and other simple sugars. All our organs and muscles use glucose as a food, and some organs—such as the brain and the kidneys—depend on a steady source of glucose to function properly.

If the pancreas, an organ located behind the stomach and near the liver, produces either no insulin or not enough, the glucose stays in the blood and doesn't make it into the cells. The cells aren't getting what they need, and over time the high levels of sugar in the bloodstream can damage a variety of organs.

Normally, the pancreas is fine-tuned to produce only the amounts of hormones the body needs at a particular time. It relies on a continual "reading" of blood glucose levels to assess, throughout the day and night, whether production levels of its hormones should be cranked up or scaled back. It's a feedback loop. If blood glucose is high—as it is after a meal—the beta cells of the pancreas are stimulated to produce more insulin. If blood glucose is lower—such as between meals or during exercise—less insulin is made. The coordinated secretion of insulin and other hormones normally maintains blood glucose levels in a tight range, providing adequate levels to those organs that require glucose.

Etiology of diabetes

Typical age ranges for the development
of diabetes

Type 1 diabetes   Type 2 diabetes

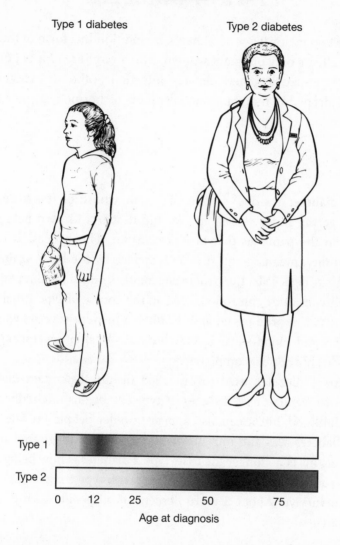

Type 1				
Type 2				
0	12	25	50	75

Age at diagnosis

Type 1 diabetes usually appears in childhood or adolescence. For reasons not entirely clear, the body's immune system attacks and destroys the cells that produce insulin. Without insulin, blood sugar levels cannot be controlled. People with type 1 diabetes must take insulin to survive.

Type 2 diabetes evolves over many years. In the early stages, this process can be reversed with dietary changes and increased physical activity. However, without enough insulin, glucose levels rise progressively. Over time, the high levels of glucose in the bloodstream can damage organs in the body.

TYPES OF DIABETES

There are two major types of diabetes, in addition to a form of the disease that affects only pregnant women. Much rarer are types of diabetes caused by specific genetic defects, infections, other diseases of the pancreas, drugs, or the abnormal secretion of hormones other than insulin.

TYPE 1

In type 1 diabetes, the body's immune system, whose job it is to destroy invading germs and diseases, attacks and destroys its own beta cells, the cells in the pancreas that produce insulin. This process is called autoimmunity, meaning an immune response by the body against itself. Without beta cells, the pancreas cannot produce insulin and glucose levels cannot be controlled. Early in the course of type 1 diabetes, the pancreas can produce enough insulin to prevent severe hyperglycemia (elevated blood sugar levels), but usually after several months production shuts down completely.

Type 1 diabetes used to be called insulin-dependent diabetes mellitus or juvenile-onset diabetes. It typically begins in childhood or young adulthood, but it can also appear in older people. At one time, type 1 diabetes was the only form of the disease diagnosed in the young, but this is no longer the case: type 2 diabetes is now being diagnosed at younger and younger ages. Those with type 1 diabetes require insulin to survive. About 5 to 10 percent of all people with diabetes have type 1.

TYPE 2

By far the most common type of diabetes, and the main focus of this book, is type 2 diabetes. This form of the disease is caused by a combination of insulin resistance and relative (not total, as in type 1) insulin deficiency. Insulin resistance means that the body's cells are not sensi-

Natural history of type 2 diabetes

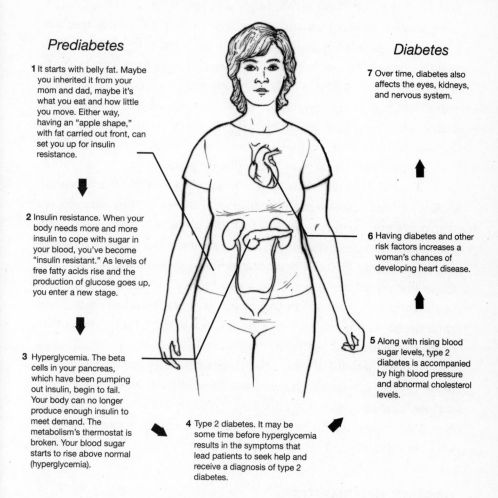

Prediabetes

1 It starts with belly fat. Maybe you inherited it from your mom and dad, maybe it's what you eat and how little you move. Either way, having an "apple shape," with fat carried out front, can set you up for insulin resistance.

2 Insulin resistance. When your body needs more and more insulin to cope with sugar in your blood, you've become "insulin resistant." As levels of free fatty acids rise and the production of glucose goes up, you enter a new stage.

3 Hyperglycemia. The beta cells in your pancreas, which have been pumping out insulin, begin to fail. Your body can no longer produce enough insulin to meet demand. The metabolism's thermostat is broken. Your blood sugar starts to rise above normal (hyperglycemia).

4 Type 2 diabetes. It may be some time before hyperglycemia results in the symptoms that lead patients to seek help and receive a diagnosis of type 2 diabetes.

Diabetes

7 Over time, diabetes also affects the eyes, kidneys, and nervous system.

6 Having diabetes and other risk factors increases a woman's chances of developing heart disease.

5 Along with rising blood sugar levels, type 2 diabetes is accompanied by high blood pressure and abnormal cholesterol levels.

When the body's cells resist the effects of insulin, the pancreas must produce increasing amounts to try to maintain normal blood glucose levels. If the pancreas cannot keep up with the demand for insulin, blood sugar levels rise and type 2 diabetes is diagnosed. Insulin resistance also plays a role in the development of cardiovascular disease (heart attacks, strokes).

tive to the effects of insulin, so that more insulin is required to maintain healthy blood sugar levels. In most people with insulin resistance, the pancreas receives signals to produce more insulin, and the beta cells compensate by making more and more insulin to maintain normal blood sugar levels. In people with insulin resistance who go on to develop diabetes, the beta cells fail to keep up with the increased demand, and blood sugar levels rise. About one-half of people with type 2 diabetes lose enough beta-cell function that they eventually need to inject insulin. Research suggests, however, that it may be preferable to start insulin injections earlier in the disease process.

Type 2 diabetes tends to run in families, but the exact genetic causes for most cases remain unclear. Numerous studies have shown that being overweight or obese and being physically inactive increase your likelihood of developing type 2 diabetes. Conversely, exercising more and eating less can delay and perhaps prevent the disease. For those who already have type 2 diabetes, these same lifestyle changes—in concert with medical control of blood sugar, blood pressure, and cholesterol—can help prevent or delay most of the complications that otherwise may occur.

About 90 to 95 percent of all cases of diabetes are type 2. It used to be called non–insulin-dependent diabetes mellitus or adult-onset diabetes, but no longer is it a disease found only in those over age forty. Nor does having type 2 as opposed to type 1 diabetes mean that you won't eventually need insulin.

GESTATIONAL DIABETES

Gestational diabetes mellitus (GDM) is a form of diabetes that develops during pregnancy. In about 3 to 5 percent of all pregnancies, a routine blood test performed between week 24 and 28 of pregnancy will reveal that a woman has gestational diabetes. A woman with gestational diabetes usually needs to modify her diet and perhaps take insulin or other medications to normalize her glucose levels and avoid harm to her baby. When medication is necessary, doctors usually prescribe

TYPES OF DIABETES

Type 1 (<10 percent of those with diabetes): An autoimmune destruction of the beta cells of the pancreas resulting in absolute insulin deficiency

Type 2 (>90 percent of those with diabetes): Progressive problem secreting insulin and meeting demands imposed by insulin resistance

Gestational diabetes (GDM): High blood sugar usually diagnosed after the twenty-fourth week of pregnancy; often resolves after delivery

Source: Adapted from the American Diabetes Association (Position Statement). Standards of Medical Care for Patients with Diabetes. *Diabetes Care,* 29 (Supplement 1) (2006): S4.

insulin, but other oral medications are also available. Many women with gestational diabetes return to normal glucose levels after pregnancy, but they have about a 50 percent chance of developing type 2 diabetes within the next five to ten years. (See Chapter 5 for more information.)

PREDIABETES: A WAKE-UP CALL

Diabetes experts have identified a stage called prediabetes when glucose levels are higher than normal but not high enough to be considered diabetes. Those with prediabetes have a very high risk of developing diabetes and are also at increased risk for cardiovascular disease. Approximately forty-one million people in the United States have prediabetes.

This is your wake-up call. Research has shown that if you take action at this stage, you can delay or possibly prevent diabetes from ever happening. We'll tell you how in Chapter 3. Unfortunately, it is also true that some of the long-term damage that occurs in diabetes, particularly damage to the heart and circulatory system, has already started in the prediabetes stage. If you have prediabetes, you are also at increased risk for heart disease and stroke.

People with prediabetes have no symptoms; the condition is dis-

covered by screening with one of the two standard blood tests for diabetes: the fasting plasma glucose (FPG) test or the oral glucose tolerance test (OGTT). The next chapter describes these tests in detail and
explains what their results mean.

People with prediabetes or diabetes are more likely to have a
cluster of risk factors for heart disease called "metabolic syndrome."
Metabolic syndrome is a package of problems that includes obesity,
prediabetes or diabetes, high blood pressure, and abnormal cholesterol
and triglycerides (another kind of fat).

IT'S AN EPIDEMIC

Diabetes, specifically type 2 diabetes, is so widespread in the United
States that it is considered an epidemic. From 1990 to 1999 there was a
41 percent increase in diagnosed cases of diabetes. More than 1.5 million new cases are now being diagnosed each year in people age twenty
and over. Although it is still primarily a disease of middle age or older,
it is increasingly being diagnosed at younger ages. The rise in diabetes
among American children and teenagers of American Indian, African
American, and Latino/Hispanic descent is an alarming problem.

We live in a society where most people drive everywhere and
shop in supermarkets rather than growing what they need to eat. Our
lifestyle often includes fast foods laden with fats. We're not as physically active as our forebears who herded sheep, hunted, and farmed.
The baby-boom generation—those born between 1946 and 1964—are
one-third of our population, and they are now middle-aged and sedentary, prime candidates for chronic diseases like type 2 diabetes.

The main culprit underlying the dramatic rise in diabetes is obesity. Not everyone with type 2 diabetes is obese, but the vast majority
are at least overweight. In fact, the incidence of diabetes in the United
States has risen steadily in tandem with the incidence of overweight
obesity, which has risen by 61 percent. More than half of all adults are

The complexion of diabetes

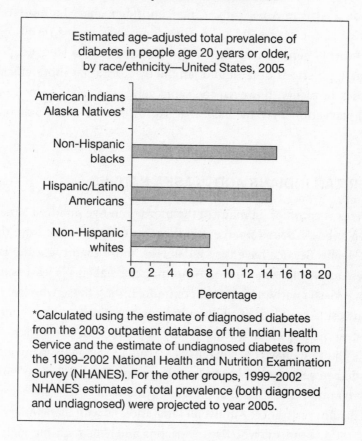

Estimated age-adjusted total prevalence of diabetes in people age 20 years or older, by race/ethnicity—United States, 2005

*Calculated using the estimate of diagnosed diabetes from the 2003 outpatient database of the Indian Health Service and the estimate of undiagnosed diabetes from the 1999–2002 National Health and Nutrition Examination Survey (NHANES). For the other groups, 1999–2002 NHANES estimates of total prevalence (both diagnosed and undiagnosed) were projected to year 2005.

In the United States type 2 diabetes is at least twice as common among women of certain ethnic subgroups than it is among whites. (National Institute of Diabetes and Digestive and Kidney Diseases, NIH.)

considered overweight or obese. Obesity rates in children have doubled and in teenagers have tripled since 1980. The epidemic of obesity has grave consequences for our health.

Diabetes is particularly prevalent in certain ethnic subgroups of Americans. Like all Americans, people in these groups have high rates of obesity and physical inactivity. In addition, they appear to carry an added genetic risk. One theory is that people with certain ethnic ancestry (some African Americans, American Indians, and Latino/Hispanic Americans, for example) have a slower metabolism as a result of a so-called thrifty gene. Their ancestors, who lived off the land, adapted to alternating periods of feast and famine by storing fat more efficiently. In times of plenty, however, the same genes that once helped people avoid starvation may increase the risk of obesity and its associated diseases.

AMERICAN INDIANS AND ALASKA NATIVES

Diabetes is common in many of the more than five hundred American Indian tribes. About 15 percent of those who receive care from the Indian Health Service have type 2 diabetes, more than twice the rate of white Americans. Among American Indians, diabetes is least common among Alaska natives and most common among those who live in the Southwest. About half of all Pima Indians ages thirty to sixty-four have diabetes, the highest frequency of any population in the world.

The Pima have been extensively studied, giving us many insights into diabetes. Scientists have identified a couple of genes—one that is more common in Pimas than in white Americans—that are associated with insulin resistance. Almost all Pima Indians with diabetes are overweight. Pima Indians who live in Arizona and eat a high-fat, high-calorie American diet have higher rates of diabetes than those living in Mexico, who are genetically thin and still eat a traditional diet low in animal fat and high in complex carbohydrates.

Type 1 diabetes, which predominantly affects people of European (particularly North European) ancestry, is very rare among American Indians. But type 2 is becoming increasingly common among American Indian children over age ten. Researchers have found that one of the strongest risk factors for diabetes in the Pima is exposure to diabetes while in the womb. One study revealed that 45 percent of women born to diabetic mothers developed diabetes by age twenty to twenty-four.

AFRICAN AMERICANS

African American women develop diabetes much more frequently than African American men in every age group. African Americans in general are almost twice as likely as white Americans to develop diabetes, and their death rates from diabetes are 27 percent higher. Nearly one out of three African American women between the ages of sixty-five and seventy-four has diabetes. Gestational diabetes is 50 to 80 percent more common in African American women than in white women, owing in part to higher levels of obesity.

Although African Americans have higher rates of obesity than whites, weight alone does not account for the disparity in diabetes rates. In fact, comparisons of the two racial groups using people with the same levels of obesity, age, and socioeconomic status still show African Americans to have a greater frequency of diabetes.

HISPANIC/LATINO AMERICANS

More Hispanic women than Hispanic men get diabetes, and both sexes are almost twice as likely to develop diabetes than are white Americans. Diabetes rates are particularly high among Mexican Americans and Puerto Ricans, though they are also high among Cuban Americans. Mexican American women, particularly if overweight, have especially high rates of gestational diabetes.

ASIAN AMERICANS AND NATIVE HAWAIIAN OR OTHER PACIFIC ISLANDERS

The data on Asian Americans and Pacific Islanders are limited, though some groups are clearly at increased risk for diabetes (Japanese, Chinese, Filipino, Korean, and Cambodian Americans). For example, 2002 data indicate that Native Hawaiians and Japanese and Filipino residents of Hawaii are twice as likely to have diabetes as are white residents of similar ages.

The complexion of America is expected to change in the upcoming decades as we increasingly become a nation of minorities. The high prevalence of diabetes in these populations is ominous, in terms of public health, costs to society, and above all the impact on individuals living with this disease.

The epidemic of diabetes is a worldwide phenomenon, affecting both developing and developed nations. But trends aren't set in stone and can be reversed.

TRUTH OR CONSEQUENCES

Everyone with diabetes or prediabetes needs to face some basic truths or deal with the consequences. This statement is meant to inspire not fear but rather a commitment. Diabetes is not destiny unless you shrug your shoulders, do nothing, and let nature take its course.

Each person finds her own way of approaching the challenge of disease. In the Navajo Indian tradition, for example, medicine men conduct sacred ceremonies to restore harmony and well-being when a person is ill. As part of one ceremony, a prayer is read encouraging the ill person to see the beauty all around her. These rituals help prepare Navajo to hear upsetting news, such as what can happen to their bodies as a result of a chronic disease like diabetes. According to Navajo belief, no situation is hopeless, and words or prayers provide reassurance that something can be done.

The message *is* hopeful. Studies have shown that the odds of developing most diabetes complications can be dramatically reduced if blood sugar levels are kept as close to normal as possible. For those of you with type 2 diabetes, this may mean changing your diet, walking more or beginning some other form of regular exercise, and taking all your prescribed medicines. For those of you with type 1, it means being extra diligent about keeping blood sugars in the normal range, with frequent blood sugar testing and adjustment of insulin doses.

Managing diabetes isn't simple, but it need not be overwhelming, either. The following list of potential complications should be an

---

CORRECTING COMMON MISCONCEPTIONS ABOUT DIABETES

- Diabetes is *not* caused by eating too many sweets (though eating too much of anything can contribute to weight gain and lead to diabetes).
- You *can* learn to give yourself injections if insulin is prescribed (it takes some getting used to but quickly becomes routine).
- You *can* eat sweets—in moderation—as part of your meal plan.
- Type 2 diabetes *is* just as serious as type 1.
- A woman with diabetes *can* have a normal, healthy baby (if she maintains blood glucose levels as close to normal as possible before and during pregnancy).
- Life as you know it is *not* over (you just have to be more mindful of your body's needs).

---

incentive to adopt healthy habits and take care of yourself. These complications do not have to be your fate. We'll talk much more about them and what you can do to reduce the risk of each in Chapter 4.

CARDIOVASCULAR (HEART) DISEASE: Heart disease, and heart attacks in particular, are the number one cause of death for women with diabetes. Diabetes erases the protection from heart disease that women usually enjoy before menopause, when menstrual periods end. The hard reality is that 65 percent of people with type 2 diabetes die of cardiovascular disease. Most of these people are obese and many have high blood pressure and cholesterol levels even before they are diagnosed with diabetes. About two-thirds of people with type 2 diabetes have high blood pressure.

STROKE: People with diabetes are two to four times more likely to suffer a stroke than the general population.

EYE DISEASE AND BLINDNESS: Diabetes is the most common cause of vision loss in adults. Each year between 12,000 and 24,000 people go blind as a result of diabetic retinopathy, a progressive eye disease affecting the eye's light-sensitive membrane, the retina, which is essential to sight.

KIDNEY DISEASE: Over time, high blood sugar levels, especially when combined with high blood pressure, damage the kidneys. When this happens, the kidneys can't perform their function of ridding the blood of waste products and extra fluid. Diabetes is the most common cause of kidney failure and accounts for 44 percent of new cases of end-stage kidney disease. In these cases, people need either dialysis (an artificial means of filtering the blood) or kidney transplantation to survive.

NEUROPATHY (NERVE DAMAGE): About 60 to 70 percent of people with diabetes have some degree of nervous system damage. This can mean numbness in the feet, slowed digestion of food, bladder control problems, or sexual dysfunction. In severe forms, nerve damage can be painful. Loss of sensation and poor blood flow to the legs and feet increase the risk of foot trauma. The most serious complication of nerve damage is a foot ulcer, which carries a high risk of infection. If a foot ulcer doesn't heal, amputation is sometimes necessary.

DENTAL DISEASE: Almost one-third of people with diabetes have severe periodontal (gum) disease. This can lead to gum recession and tooth loss.

A MESSAGE OF HOPE

Never before has diabetes affected so many people. But never before have we had so many tools to manage it. We now know that the long-term complications can be prevented or delayed through tight control of blood sugar levels and lifestyle changes. Recent studies have also shown that type 2 diabetes, which is currently an epidemic, is not inevitable. It can be prevented.

For type 1 diabetes, the next gold ring we'd like to grab is a cure or a way to prevent the disease from ever developing. For type 2 diabetes, the big pay-off would be to put effective, preventive measures into widespread practice to halt the epidemic. If you have prediabetes, that advance could start with you.

2

Diagnosis

Betty has just found out that she has diabetes and is feeling overwhelmed. Her physician told her she needs to lose weight, exercise more, and learn how to monitor her glucose levels at home. She has tried to lose weight in the past but has never been successful. She can't imagine how she'll meet these new challenges while caring for her two young children.

The symptoms can be barely noticeable or not noticeable at all. But because undiagnosed diabetes can have serious consequences, it is extremely important that you get tested at the first suspicion of a problem. Even without any of the symptoms we list below, women who are older than forty-five or who have one or more risk factors for diabetes should be screened. Testing for the disease should be a routine part of health maintenance, like having a mammogram or a PAP smear. The tests for diabetes screening and for diagnosis are the same.

The earlier you know you have the disease the better. Someone with undiagnosed diabetes does not know she is at risk for eye, kidney, and nerve damage, as well as heart disease and stroke, and therefore can't lower her risk. She doesn't know she has an extra incentive to lose weight and follow a healthier lifestyle. A newly diagnosed woman who has not been screened regularly has probably had diabetes for five to ten years and has already begun to develop complications.

In the past, type 1 diabetes, not type 2, was associated with most complications. But because people are getting type 2 diabetes at an earlier age and living longer with the disease, they too are developing complications associated with long-term exposure to high glucose levels.

Knowing is the first step toward preventing complications. As frightening as it is to hear that something might be wrong with you, imagine how much more upsetting it would be to live with additional problems that might have been avoided. An added bonus to knowing is that you can help your whole family lower their risk as well.

SYMPTOMS

The symptoms of type 1 and type 2 diabetes can be nearly the same. The most significant difference is that the symptoms of type 1 tend to come on quickly and more dramatically. Women who have type 2 diabetes may not notice the symptoms because they develop more slowly or not at all.

The following symptoms can be signs of diabetes, though only proper testing can tell for sure. See your physician if you experience any of them regularly:

→ increased frequency and volume of urination. You may notice that you can no longer sleep through the night without getting up to use the bathroom.

→ unquenchable thirst

➡ dehydration, indicated by dry lips and sunken eyes

➡ extreme hunger. Some people will even lose weight despite eating more.

➡ fatigue

➡ blurry eyesight

➡ headaches

➡ cuts and sores that heal slowly

➡ numbness or tingling in the hands or feet

➡ chronic yeast infections or new or frequent urinary tract infections

Many of these symptoms result from the abnormally high level of glucose in the blood and urine that is the hallmark of diabetes.

Sometimes type 1 diabetes is diagnosed in a crisis situation called "ketoacidosis." When insulin levels drop very low, fat stores start dissolving, which is what happens when someone is starving. This process produces waste products called ketones, which leave the body in a highly acidic and dangerously out-of-balance state. Symptoms of ketoacidosis include nausea, vomiting, or stomach pains; labored or rapid breathing; and fruity-smelling breath. If you have these symptoms, call

---

DIAGNOSING DIABETES

The following factors must be present for a diagnosis of diabetes:

• Any combination of these symptoms: excessive thirst or hunger, frequent urination, unexplained fatigue, weight loss, or frequent infections with a random blood glucose greater than or equal to 200 mg/dl. Certain symptoms such as headaches, confusion, irritability, and depression may occur more frequently in those with hyperglycemia.

• Laboratory tests (require confirmation)

  –Fasting blood glucose greater than or equal to 126 mg/dl

  –A two-hour blood glucose greater than or equal to 200 mg/dl on an Oral Glucose Tolerance Test (OGTT)

Source: Adapted from American Diabetes Association (Position Statement). Standards of Medical Care for Patients with Diabetes. Diabetes Care, 29 (Supplement 1) (2006): S5.

---

your health care provider immediately. We'll talk more about ketoacidosis in Chapter 4.

RISKY BUSINESS

Women with known risk factors for diabetes should be particularly vigilant for signs of the disease. Risk factors are characteristics that appear to be associated with a disease. They might include personal behavior or lifestyle, environmental exposure, or an inherited trait that scientific evidence has associated with a disease. Having one or more risk factors increases your chance of developing a disease but does not mean you will definitely get it. On the other hand, not having a risk factor for a disease doesn't mean you are home free—it simply means that your likelihood of developing it is not high.

Risk factors for type 2 diabetes include:

➡ being overweight or obese, particularly if the weight is centered around the abdomen. Refer to the body mass index (BMI) table in Appendix 1 to determine if you are normal weight, overweight, or obese. Overweight is defined as having a BMI of 25 or greater; obesity is indicated by a BMI of 30 or greater. The higher your BMI, the greater your risk for diabetes.

➡ age forty-five or older

➡ family background that is African American, American Indian, Hispanic American, Asian American, or Pacific Islander

➡ family history of type 2 diabetes, such as a parent, brother, or sister with the disease

➡ inactive lifestyle, defined as walking or exercising fewer than three times a week

➡ high blood pressure, currently defined as 140/90 or higher. Blood pressure measures the force of blood against the artery walls: the pressure as the heart beats (systolic)/ the pressure as the heart relaxes between beats (diastolic).

➡ cholesterol and/or triglyceride levels that are not normal. The choles-

terol number that is most frequently abnormal in people with diabetes
or at risk for the disease is the HDL (the so-called good cholesterol),
which in women at risk for diabetes is 40 or lower (35 or lower in
men). You are also at risk if your triglyceride level is 250 mg/dl or
greater. Triglycerides are fats that circulate in the bloodstream along
with cholesterol and are stored in the body's fatty tissue, for example,
around the waist and hips.

➡ history of gestational diabetes or having delivered a baby that weighed
more than nine pounds

➡ impaired glucose tolerance (IGT) or impaired fasting glucose (also
called prediabetes) on a previous test. (We'll describe scores that indicate prediabetes and put you at risk later in this chapter.)

➡ certain other endocrine conditions (disorders of the pituitary gland,
adrenal gland, and ovaries, for example, and the hormones they produce), such as polycystic ovary syndrome (PCOS), also increase risk
substantially. We'll discuss PCOS in Chapter 5.

The current recommendation is that everyone age forty-five and
older should be screened for diabetes. If the result is normal, you
should be retested every three years. If you are at higher risk, with one
or more of the factors listed above, annual testing is suggested. Some
experts think that screening should start at an even younger age for

WHO SHOULD BE SCREENED FOR DIABETES?

All women over forty-five should be screened. If the result is normal, repeat
the test every three years. Get a screening test earlier and annually if you
have any of these risk factors:

• you have prediabetes
• you are overweight or obese
• you have a parent, brother, or sister with type 2 diabetes
• you are a member of a high-risk ethnic group
• you had a baby who weighed more than nine pounds at birth or you had
gestational diabetes
• you have high blood pressure
• you have abnormal cholesterol or triglyceride levels
• you have polycystic ovary syndrome (PCOS)

those with one or more risk factors, particularly if their body mass index is greater than 25, or if their ethnicity puts them in the high-risk category.

CHILDREN AT RISK

Type 2 diabetes is increasing in children and adolescents, particularly among African Americans, Hispanic Americans, and American Indians. If you are at risk, your children or grandchildren probably are, too. This is especially true if they are overweight.

About 90 percent of children with type 2 diabetes have dark, rough patches of skin on their necks or armpits. Called acanthosis nigricans, these patches indicate that insulin levels are high and that insulin resistance is present. The American Diabetes Association (ADA) considers children and adolescents at "substantial risk" if they are overweight with two of the following risk factors:

- family history of diabetes
- member of a high-risk ethnic group
- signs of insulin resistance, such as hypertension, high cholesterol, polycystic ovary syndrome, or acanthosis nigricans

Some evidence suggests that low-birthweight babies who were not born prematurely are at an increased risk for type 2 diabetes. Low birthweight not associated with prematurity indicates that the fetus grew slowly for some reason. Small size at birth combined with obesity later in life appears to increase one's risk of developing type 2 diabetes.

Children who are at substantial risk for type 2 diabetes should be screened after age ten, or earlier if puberty starts earlier.

There are blood tests available to identify children at higher risk for developing type 1 diabetes, but they are not routinely done. Since there are no effective methods to prevent type 1 diabetes, widespread screening is not recommended. Prevention studies are currently look-

---

CHILDREN SHOULD BE SCREENED FOR TYPE 2 DIABETES IF:

- they are overweight (their doctor says their weight places them above the 85th percentile for age and height), and
- they have at least two risk factors:
  - –family history of type 2 diabetes in first- or second-degree relatives
  - –member of high-risk ethnic group
  - –conditions associated with insulin resistance: hypertension, hyperlipidemia (abnormal cholesterol panel), polycystic ovary syndrome (PCOS)
  - –maternal history of GDM

Testing should begin at age ten or at onset of puberty, whichever comes first, and then be repeated every two years with fasting blood glucose.

Source: Adapted from American Diabetes Association (Position Statement). Standards of Medical Care for Patients with Diabetes. *Diabetes Care,* 29 (Supplement 1) (2006): S6.

---

ing at ways to affect the body's immune system to prevent beta-cell destruction before insulin production shuts down. Some studies have been promising, but thus far nothing has led to the Holy Grail, a cure for type 1 diabetes.

Risk factors for type 1 diabetes in children include:

➡ a parent, brother, or sister with type 1 diabetes. The risk is slightly higher if the parent with diabetes is the father as opposed to the mother. A family history of type 2 diabetes is not a risk factor for type 1.

➡ presence of another autoimmune disorder, such as Graves disease, Hashimoto's thyroiditis, or Addison's disease

TAKE THE TEST

Perhaps your symptoms brought you to your doctor's office, or more likely, maybe you or your doctor raised the issue of risk factors for diabetes during a routine visit (remember that type 2 diabetes is most often a silent disease with few or no symptoms). Your doctor will measure your blood pressure and weight, and ask you questions about your symptoms and family history of diabetes, your diet and exercise patterns, and any history of cigarette smoking. She may then order a fasting cholesterol and other lipid tests. And, of course, she'll order the definitive test for diabetes itself—one simple blood test.

Diabetes and prediabetes are both diagnosed by how much glucose (sugar) is in your blood. There are three ways to test blood glucose levels: fasting plasma glucose (FPG), oral glucose tolerance test (OGTT), or a random plasma glucose test. Prediabetes can be diagnosed only by the FPG or OGTT.

Note that the concentration of glucose in the blood is indicated in the United States by mg/dl (milligrams/deciliter); elsewhere in the world, it is measured in mmol/l (millimoles/liter). You may see it expressed both ways.

RANDOM PLASMA GLUCOSE TEST

The random plasma glucose test is a nonfasting test, meaning you don't need to abstain from food and drink before blood is drawn. Sometimes suspected cases of diabetes turn up during a routine physical exam when blood is drawn for other tests. If someone with obvious symptoms of diabetes has a random plasma glucose concentration greater than or equal to 200 mg/dl (11.1 mmol/l), she probably has diabetes. To make sure, her doctor will order a fasting test or a hemoglobin A_{1c} test, which we describe a little later in this chapter.

FASTING PLASMA GLUCOSE (FPG)

An FPG test is performed after fasting; the patient may not have anything to eat or drink except water for at least eight hours before the blood is drawn. The American Diabetes Association and its panel of medical experts have recommended the FPG as their first choice for general screening for diabetes. The exception is when testing for gestational diabetes and in follow-up tests for women who had gestational diabetes. Then an OGTT (see below) is done.

A normal FPG is up to 100 mg/dl (5.6 mmol/l). An FPG in the range of 100 mg/dl to 125 mg/dl (5.6 to 6.9 mmol/l) is considered impaired fasting glucose, which is one type of prediabetes. A person with prediabetes is at risk for developing diabetes and should begin to make

What the test scores mean

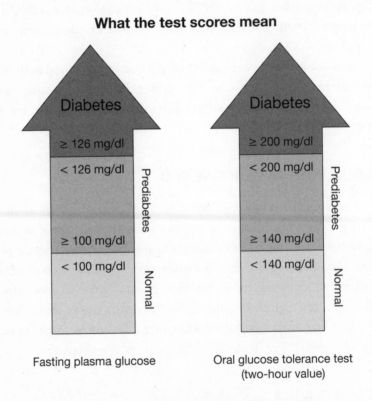

Fasting plasma glucose

Oral glucose tolerance test
(two-hour value)

Almost all people who eventually develop type 2 diabetes first go through a prediabetes phase. The development of type 2 diabetes is usually a gradual progression. The values that determine whether your plasma glucose level is normal, prediabetic, or diabetic differs according to which test is used. (American Diabetes Association.)

lifestyle changes to try to prevent it. Diabetes is diagnosed when FPG is 126 mg/dl (7 mmol/l) or higher on two different days.

ORAL GLUCOSE TOLERANCE TEST (OGTT)

The OGTT is performed after an overnight fast of at least eight hours. First, blood is drawn to establish the FPG, then the patient is given seventy-five grams of a glucose solution—a sugary cola-like syrup— to drink. A second blood sample is obtained two hours after the glucose solution is taken. This "stress test" for diabetes determines how the person's body handles a large dose of extra glucose. The OGTT is the most sensitive test for detecting diabetes and predi- abetes.

In people without diabetes, blood sugar increases somewhat af- ter drinking the glucose solution, peaks after one hour, and then de- creases. A normal two-hour value is less than 140 mg/dl (7.8 mmol/l).

In IGT (impaired glucose tolerance), the two-hour blood sugar level is between 140 and 199 mg/dl (7.8 to 11.1 mmol/l). IGT increases your risk for diabetes and heart disease. Recent research has indicated that IGT appears to be a stronger predictor of diabetes and heart dis- ease than impaired fasting glucose. A person with IGT should begin lifestyle changes, consider medications for diabetes and heart disease prevention, and be retested for diabetes annually.

Diabetes is diagnosed when the two-hour blood sugar value is 200 mg/dl (11.1 mmol/l) or higher. This indicates that glucose is not being metabolized as it should be. This finding needs to be confirmed by repeating the oral glucose tolerance test.

The OGTT is also used to screen pregnant women for gesta- tional diabetes, which almost always has no symptoms. Parts of the procedure—such as the amount of the sugary syrup you drink—are slightly different when testing for GDM as opposed to type 2, as are the values that indicate a problem. We describe the diagnosis and treat- ment of GDM in Chapter 5.

WHICH TEST IS BEST?

The purpose of screening people who have no symptoms is to identify those with diabetes or prediabetes as early as possible so they can start correcting their abnormal sugar levels. The cut-off points of normal and diabetic glucose levels are based on the levels associated with diabetes-specific complications, like diabetic eye disease.

There has been considerable controversy about which test, the FPG or OGTT, is best for diagnosing diabetes. The American Diabetes Association recommends the FPG as the primary diagnostic test, mainly because it is more convenient and less expensive than the OGTT.

But some diabetes experts are concerned that by using only the FPG test we may miss many people who are at risk. It is now clear that those with impaired glucose tolerance (which the OGTT measures) are at a higher risk for developing cardiovascular complications than those with impaired fasting glucose (diagnosed with the FPG). Impaired glucose tolerance and impaired fasting glucose may even be two distinct forms of prediabetes. Finally, the OGTT diagnoses women with diabetes more sensitively than does the fasting test.

Until the controversy regarding fasting and oral glucose tolerance testing is resolved, however, our advice is to do the fasting screening. If you or your doctor think you are at a particularly high risk, then you should do the OGTT instead.

One alternative being discussed is the possibility of diagnosing diabetes with a combination of a fasting glucose test and the hemoglobin A_{1c} (described below), which is currently used to assess how well someone with diabetes is maintaining her blood sugar levels over time.

THE HEMOGLOBIN A_{1c} (HgbA$_{1c}$)

The HgbA$_{1c}$ test is like a snapshot of your glucose levels for the past two to three months. Whereas the FPG and OGTT measure glucose levels at specific times during the day, the HgbA$_{1c}$ test (also known as glycohemoglobin) reflects the average of all glucose levels over the previous two to three months. The HgbA₁c test measures the fraction of hemoglobin molecules (which carry oxygen and make red blood cells red) that have glucose attached to them. The glucose that sticks to the hemoglobin will stay attached for the lifecycle of the red blood cell (about 120 days).

No fasting is necessary for the HgbA₁c test, and the blood sample can be taken at any time of day. A score of 4 to 6 percent is normal for people without diabetes. Any level above 6 percent is abnormal, and the higher the level of HgbA₁c, the higher the average blood sugars have been in the past two to three months (see Table 2.1). Current recom-

Table 2.1   What blood glucose scores mean

Target goals for A_{1c} (%)	
Level of control	A_{1c}
Normal	less than 6
Goal	less than 7
Take action	7 or more

How A_{1c} corresponds to blood glucose testing	
A_{1c} level (%)	Blood glucose test average (mg/dl)
12	300
11	270
10	240
9	210
8	180
7	150
6	120
5	80

Target goals for blood glucose levels in nonpregnant women	
Testing time	Plasma or fingerstick values
Before meals	80–120
1–2 hours after meals	less than 180
At bedtime	100–140

Source: Adapted from "Know Your Blood Sugar Numbers," National Diabetes Education Program (www.ndep.nih.gov/diabetes/pubs/KnowNumbers_Eng.pdf).

mendations are to lower HbA$_{1c}$ to as close to the nondiabetic range as possible, with less than 7 percent being a practical goal that will effectively decrease the development and progression of eye, kidney, and nerve complications.

WHY ME?

It can be overwhelming to hear that you have a disease for which there is no cure. If you've just been told you have diabetes, you probably have many questions: Am I going to need injections of insulin? Can I still eat my favorite foods? Can I have children? Will they be at risk for diabetes? Will I still be attractive to my partner? Am I going to be a burden to my family? You will find answers to these and many more questions in this book and from people and resources your physician can recommend. But there's one message we want you to hear loud and clear: Diabetes should not stop you from doing anything in life you want to do.

> Diabetes should not stop you from doing anything in life you want to do.

If you've been diagnosed with diabetes, you may have found that you have one or more of the risk factors listed earlier. That may, in part, answer the question, "Why me?" No one, however, can answer the more spiritual aspect of this question. Some people seem to be at much higher risk than others and yet they don't get diabetes. We don't know what protects them and didn't protect you.

We are beginning to understand how people with risk factors might prevent the disease, and for them the next chapter is devoted to prevention. But if you have already been diagnosed with diabetes, you obviously can't prevent the disease. You *can* reduce your chances of developing complications. You *can* control what you do from this day forward.

This is not to minimize the shock of being diagnosed with diabetes. Many people don't feel at all sick or even different when diagnosed, which only adds to their feelings of disbelief. Some need to process their shock and go through stages of grief: denial that they really have a problem, anger, fear, sadness or depression, and finally acceptance. The roller coaster of emotions you may be experiencing is very normal. Like everyone else, you will have ups and downs. Periods of sadness are inevitable, and at such times it's crucial that you reach out to family, friends, and professionals to help you cope. We'll discuss other strategies for dealing with stress and sadness in Chapter 6.

We have found that the people with diabetes who do best are those who are able to learn new strategies for adjusting to necessary lifestyle changes. They approach their lives with optimism and view challenges as surmountable. They are willing to do the work necessary to have a healthy life. They have created a supportive community that often includes family, friends, and neighbors.

Granted, you now have a lot to learn, but information can be absorbed gradually in manageable portions. Changes don't have to be made overnight. You can make them in slow, incremental steps. For many of you, it may take as long as six months to make the rounds to the various medical specialists, diabetes nurse educators, and dietitians who will help you understand the effects of diet, exercise, and medications, and to develop a treatment plan that works for you. New tools and devices make it easier than ever to measure blood sugar levels and administer medications. Diabetes classes and support groups can be found in most communities. Your health care team can direct you to resources that will give you the best chance of coping successfully with your disease. (See Chapter 8 for a list of resources.) You don't have to manage alone.

Table 2.2 gives you a sense of what a typical day is like for a woman with diabetes.

A PARTNERSHIP WITH YOUR MEDICAL PROVIDERS

Most likely your primary care physician diagnosed your diabetes. Diabetes is so common now that all general practitioners (also called internists or family practitioners) have experience with it. Ideally,

Table 2.2 A day in the life of a woman with diabetes

Before diabetes	After diagnosis
Morning: Wake up, have breakfast of coffee with cream and sugar	Wake up, test blood sugar, take your medications with breakfast as directed by treatment team; have your coffee with soy or skim milk, with or without artificial sweetener
Mealtimes: Eat meals at irregular times, relying on fast food, food from vending machines, take-out, snacks	Test blood sugar (if you adjust your insulin based on blood sugar levels), take diabetes medications as directed by treatment team; monitor what and how much you eat, emphasizing whole grains, lean proteins, "good" fats, and fresh produce, all with the aim of avoiding blood sugar spikes
Cooking at home: Cook food in margarine; eat bread and baked goods high in trans fat, sugar, not much fiber	Switch to good fats such as olive oil; reduce reliance on added sweeteners; switch to whole grains and dark leafy greens; try new combinations: whole wheat pasta doesn't go well with tomato but tastes fine with pesto
Food shopping: Shop while hungry, loading cart with frozen dinners, snacking in the check-out line	Shop after a meal or small snack; follow a list; choose foods for high-fiber, low-sugar content, and check carefully for trans fats; read labels carefully: some fruit yogurts have more sugar per serving than a bowl of Count Chocula cereal
Work: 4 P.M. visit to the candy machine; doughnuts brought in by co-workers	Monitor blood sugar at work; keep healthy snacks on hand in your desk; lobby for healthy choices in the office machines; instead of the doughnuts, bring in a healthier, homemade coffeecake you know you can eat
Exercise: Sporadic attempts to get an exercise program started, but just too busy or tired	Make a commitment to exercise four times a week; find short, safe walks near your home; purchase small hand weights to use while watching TV; find an exercise class for comradeship. Hate the gym? Try indoor rock-climbing or belly dancing; learn how to exercise safely and recognize warning signs of hypoglycemia; adjust meals and insulin to accommodate your new level of activity
Social events: Holiday traditions built around sweet treats or watching college football games; after-work visits to the local bar	Learn to check your diet, monitor glucose, and stick to your plan even when you're around family and old friends; suggest a walk after Thanksgiving dinner; start a new after-work tradition that doesn't include happy hour at a bar; ask about health-club membership refunds or rebates offered through your work

Table 2.2 *(continued)*

Before diabetes	After diagnosis
Sleep:	
Stay up late snacking in front of the TV, fall into bed late, and sleep poorly	Remember to perform home blood glucose fingersticks and eat a pre-bedtime snack if indicated; try yoga and meditation to relax
Foot care:	
Examine feet only when you get a splinter	After your shower and before bed, examine your feet carefully for injury and ulcers; make sure you have shoes that fit properly and protect your feet; if you always stub your toe on a certain piece of furniture, move the furniture!

After diagnosis, your days will also include:
• going to follow-up medical appointments three to four times a year
• taking your medications consistently at home every day
• gathering information on your health for your next medical visit
• going to education classes to learn more about diabetes
• doing what you need to do to prevent medical complications associated with diabetes

everyone with diabetes should have an interdisciplinary team of health care professionals to help manage her care. The reality is that outside of urban areas, there are fewer specialists, so primary care physicians and nurse practitioners usually take on the role of at least some of these professionals. Specialists are usually consulted as needed.

PHYSICIAN

Your primary care physician may manage your treatment, especially if you have type 2 diabetes, or you may want to see a physician who specializes in diabetes. Most people with type 1 diabetes see an endocrinologist, a doctor who specializes in problems of the body's glands and hormones. Diabetologists are endocrinologists who have a special focus on the care of people with diabetes. Many of them are certified by the American Diabetes Association (see the list of references at the end of Chapter 8).

YOUR PARTNERS IN HEALTH

- Primary care physician (internist or family practitioner) or nurse practitioner
- Endocrinologist or diabetologist
- Certified diabetes nurse educator
- Registered dietitian
- Exercise specialist
- Ophthalmologist (for an eye examination)
- Podiatrist (to check your feet)
- Dentist (to check for tooth decay and gum disease)
- Obstetrician with experience in high-risk pregnancy (if you are currently pregnant or planning a pregnancy)
- Behaviorist (could be a health coach, psychologist, social worker, or psychiatrist)

DIABETES NURSE EDUCATOR

After your diagnosis, your physician may have referred you to a diabetes nurse educator, usually a registered nurse or nurse practitioner who has expertise or certification in diabetes care. This person is a teacher, a motivator, a guiding hand, and a constant source of advice. She or he will teach you how to manage your diabetes yourself on a day-to-day basis, including monitoring your blood glucose levels, giving injections if needed, modifying your diet and physical activity, and helping you to coordinate all these tasks with your usual activities.

DIETITIAN

A registered dietitian, or RD, can help you make necessary changes in your diet and lifestyle. She may help you plan meals and coordinate your medication schedule with meals. Her job is to help you adjust your shopping, cooking, and eating to make your diet healthier. If you are overweight, she will help you understand where the excess calories

WHAT YOU LEARN AT DIABETES EDUCATION CLASSES

* How to understand, organize, and take your medications
* How to monitor your blood glucose at home
* How to design a meal plan
* How to deal with emergencies, like low blood sugar or a sick day
* How to prevent and treat acute and chronic complications of diabetes
* How to network and ensure psychosocial support
* How to plan and get through pregnancy safely for you and your baby

are coming from and how to reduce them. She will teach you the effects of specific types of food on glucose levels. She will work on meal plans that take into account your tastes (your ethnicity and cooking style, for example), the amount of time your lifestyle allows you to prepare meals, and other shopping, cooking, and eating habits.

Today the thinking is that you don't have to change your lifestyle to adapt to your medication schedule; your medication schedule should accommodate your meal habits. If you always eat dinner at 7 P.M., for example, your medications, and especially insulin, will be timed accordingly. Insulin comes in very-rapid and rapid-acting, intermediate-acting, and long-acting forms that can be adjusted to suit all sorts of work, school, and leisure schedules.

OTHER SPECIALISTS

You may be referred to other medical specialists to screen for or treat any complications related to diabetes. You will probably be sent to an eye specialist (ophthalmologist), or in some cases an optometrist, after your diagnosis and usually every year thereafter. If you develop or are at risk for foot problems, you may be referred to a podiatrist. You may need to see a cardiologist to help you prevent or treat heart disease. A nephrologist, a kidney specialist, may be consulted if you develop kidney disease. Sometimes it helps to see a mental health professional—a psychologist, psychiatrist, or social worker—if you're having difficulty adjusting to the disease and its management.

Don't be afraid to ask questions. We recommend that you make a list of questions before your appointments, when you are less nervous and have time to think. Your health care providers are busy people, but they are there to help you.

All this talk of managing and adjusting to diabetes may seem restrictive. But once your medical team has helped you put together a plan that fits with the demands of your life, you will find that diabetes isn't nearly as restrictive or oppressive as you feared. Gradually, diabetes care becomes routine, like brushing your teeth. Diabetes can't currently be cured, but with your determination it can be controlled.

3

Prevention

Susan has always struggled with her weight. She had gestational diabetes during her last pregnancy and has been told she is at risk for developing type 2 diabetes. Despite feeling frustrated many days, she has lost ten pounds in four months after joining a weight-loss program and starting to walk to work instead of driving. Susan is determined to continue losing weight because she does not want to develop diabetes.

You obviously can't turn back time and change your age. Nor can you alter your race, ethnicity, and genes. But there are some things you *can* change to reduce your risk of developing diabetes. In this chapter we will talk more in-depth about who is at risk for developing type 2 diabetes, what risk means, and how we know diabetes can be prevented. We will also provide some easy-to-follow strategies to help women from all walks of life prevent diabetes through positive lifestyle changes. If you succeed, this may be the only chapter in this book you'll need.

Even if you've just been diagnosed with diabetes, you can still put this chapter to good use. We can help motivate you to follow a healthier lifestyle. You, in turn, can help your children, grandchildren, sisters, mother, aunts, husband, partners, and friends do the same.

When we talk about preventing diabetes, we are referring to type 2 diabetes. At this point type 1 cannot be prevented. Researchers are hard at work searching for ways to stop or delay the beta-cell destruction that leads to type 1 diabetes. For example, one research trial sought to determine if low doses of insulin started early in those at high risk would prevent the disease. Unfortunately, those who took preventative insulin were no better off than those who did not. Other experiments have also been disappointing, delaying the further destruction of beta-cells for only brief periods of time; however, some promising approaches remain to be tested. If you have prediabetes or are at risk for developing type 2 diabetes, the picture is not as bleak, and you can take action to prevent the disease.

A FORMULA FOR HEALTH

We have conclusive evidence that by making fairly modest changes to your diet and level of physical activity, you can prevent or at least delay the onset of diabetes. The Diabetes Prevention Program (DPP), a national clinical trial we'll describe later, found that just thirty minutes a day of moderate-intensity physical activity combined with a 5 to 10 percent loss in body weight will reduce a person's risk of getting diabetes by more than one-half (by 58 percent, to be precise). This was true for all participants in the study, regardless of sex, age, or ethnic group. For many, blood glucose levels returned to normal. Researchers also tested metformin, a medication used to treat type 2 diabetes, to see if it also worked as a preventative. The results were encouraging, but not nearly as impressive as changes in diet and physical activity.

We keep saying that the disease can be prevented "or at least delayed" because the DPP followed participants only for an average of about three years. This was enough time to see how remarkable the results were. It could very well be that if we followed those same people the rest of their lives, and if they maintained their lifestyle changes, they would never get diabetes. The original participants in the Diabetes Prevention Program are still being followed to see if this is true.

We do know from other studies, however, that most people with prediabetes will develop type 2 diabetes in ten years if they do nothing. In addition, over time many of them will develop the complications of diabetes, which will certainly affect the quality of their lives. Who wants to take the chance that this will happen to them?

Before you roll your eyes and say that dieting has never worked for you, let us explain what a 5 to 10 percent weight loss means. For a woman who weighs 175 pounds, for example, a 5 percent weight loss is 8.75 pounds; 10 percent is 17.5 pounds. The DPP aimed for a weight loss of at least 7 percent, so figure the minimum you would need to lose by multiplying your weight in pounds times .07. That number is your target weight loss.

This figure may not put you at your "ideal" weight, but it is a reasonable target for preventing type 2 diabetes. Evidence shows that weight loss, particularly as a result of eating less fatty foods, may also reduce your chances of developing heart disease and certain cancers, such as breast and colon cancer.

Now for the other part of the equation. We use the words "physical activity" to avoid the often-dreaded "e" word: "exercise." You don't

---

YOUR TARGET WEIGHT LOSS

[Your current weight] times either 0.05 (5 percent loss) or 0.10 (10 percent loss) = sufficient weight loss to reduce your risk of developing diabetes by 50 percent.

So, for example, if you weigh 200 pounds:

200 × 0.05 = 10 pounds; 200 × 0.10 = 20 pounds. You need to lose between 10 and 20 pounds to increase the odds of preventing diabetes.

have to run a marathon to prevent diabetes. In the Diabetes Prevention Program, positive results required only thirty minutes of moderately strenuous activity five days a week. Walking briskly is a great way to increase physical activity, but it is by no means the only way. Numerous other activities also fall into this category. But we'll get to that.

WHO IS AT RISK?

In the last chapter we listed risk factors for diabetes. Those same factors place you at risk for prediabetes. Prediabetes means that your blood glucose levels are higher than normal but not yet high enough to be considered diabetes. People with prediabetes are extremely likely to go on to develop type 2 diabetes.

Take the following quiz to see if you might be at risk for developing prediabetes and diabetes. If you check off one or more of these statements, you are at risk. In addition, risk goes up with age, particularly after age forty-five.

( ) My BMI is 25 or greater (see BMI table, Appendix 1).
( ) I have a parent, brother, or sister with type 2 diabetes.
( ) I am African American, American Indian, Asian American, Hispanic, or Pacific Islander.
( ) I have had gestational diabetes or have given birth to a baby that weighed nine pounds or more.
( ) I have been told that I have high blood pressure, or my blood pressure is 140/90 or higher.
( ) My cholesterol and/or triglyceride levels are not normal. My HDL (the so-called good cholesterol) is 50 or lower and/or my triglyceride level is 250 mg/dl or greater. (Triglycerides are fats that circulate in the bloodstream along with cholesterol.)
( ) I am fairly inactive. I exercise fewer than two times a week.

If you think you are at risk, talk to your physician at your next annual physical. Request one of the blood glucose tests described in

---

CALCULATING BODY MASS INDEX (BMI)

To calculate your BMI, divide your weight in pounds by your height (in inches) squared, then multiply that number by 703. For example, if you are 5′4″ and weigh 125 lbs.:

125 ÷ (64 × 64) × 703 = 21

< 18.5 = underweight

≥ 25 = overweight

≥ 30 = obese

Chapter 2. The idea of preventing diabetes is relatively new to physicians as well as to the public, so you might have to broach the subject.

Prediabetes is not just a warning of diabetes. Someone with blood sugars in the prediabetes range is also 1.5 times more likely to have cardiovascular disease, even if she never develops type 2 diabetes. There is evidence that the same strategies that help prevent diabetes, specifically, eating less fat, losing weight, and becoming more active, will, when combined with medication to lower blood pressure and cholesterol (if prescribed), help prevent heart disease as well.

THE RISK IS REAL

Changing your lifestyle is difficult. We understand perfectly well that no one will undertake change unless she believes the risk to her health is real. It's human nature to appreciate the general concept of risk—such as that overweight people over age forty-five are at risk of developing type 2 diabetes—but to think that it won't happen to you. But if you have one or more of the risk factors listed above, diabetes *can* happen to you.

Research on risk perception, however, has shown that our fears do not always match the facts. In the wake of a terrorist attack, for example, people greatly fear another one. Especially in the immediate aftermath, the risk *feels* very real. Yet it is far more likely that any one of us will die in a car accident, particularly if we don't wear a seat belt, than in a terrorist attack. Yet chances are we have all spent more time worrying about a terrorist attack than about an automobile accident.

Our point is to contrast this very remote risk with one that is all too real: the risk factors for diabetes are based on strong scientific evidence. We don't just feel there's a risk; we *know* there's one. Although being at risk does not mean that you will definitely get diabetes, many scientific studies reveal that there is a greater chance that you will.

Moreover, whereas fear of terrorism leaves people feeling helpless, the threat of diabetes need not. The risk is real, but you can lower it by taking concrete steps. This is true no matter how many risk factors you may have.

THE EVIDENCE

Several clinical trials have shown that the progress from prediabetes to diabetes is not inevitable provided that you change how you live your life. Clinical trials are research studies designed to produce statistically valid information about how best to treat patients. Since the 1940s, when a large clinical trial established the effectiveness of the antibiotic streptomycin in treating tuberculosis, clinical trials have become the primary way we develop and objectively evaluate new treatments.

Clinical trials have played a critical role in improving diabetes treatment and the prevention of its complications. Ineffective treatments have been discontinued. The more effective ones have improved the length and quality of life for people with diabetes. A cure may someday come from clinical trials.

In the meantime, we now have dramatic, consistent evidence from several well-designed clinical trials that we can prevent type 2 diabetes. Earlier studies from around the world had suggested that changing diet and physical activity might prevent type 2 diabetes. But two later studies, reported in 2001 and 2002, provided proof. Both studies utilized a control group, that is, participants in the study who did not receive the treatment whose effectiveness was being assessed. Control groups tell us whether the treatment being studied is better than a current treatment or better than doing nothing.

THE FINNISH DIABETES PREVENTION STUDY

The first study, conducted in Finland, consisted of 522 middle-aged overweight adults (mostly women) with prediabetes. The Finnish Diabetes Prevention Study found that participants could reduce their risk of type 2 diabetes by 58 percent with modest weight loss (about seven pounds, or about 5 percent of body weight), improved diet (less fat, more fiber), and increased physical activity (moderate exercise thirty minutes a day). The group that received individualized counseling on nutrition, weight control, and physical activity met with a counselor seven times in the first year of the study and then every three months for the next three years. The results of this lifestyle intervention group were compared with the results in the control group. The findings were reported in the May 3, 2001, issue of the *New England Journal of Medicine.*

THE DIABETES PREVENTION PROGRAM

The second major study was even larger, consisting of 3,234 overweight men and women in the United States with prediabetes. Like the Finnish study, the Diabetes Prevention Program also found a 58 percent reduction in the risk of type 2 diabetes through lifestyle changes. Approximately two-thirds of the study participants were women. In addition, about 45 percent of participants were from minority groups that are at particularly high risk of developing type 2 diabetes: American Indians, African Americans, Hispanic Americans, Asian Americans, and Pacific Islanders.

In the DPP all participants were told to follow a healthy lifestyle by eating less fat, exercising more, and giving up cigarettes, but one group received intensive training in diet, exercise, and lifestyle modification (for example, how to shop for and cook healthier meals and overcome personal obstacles to losing weight). The goal of those in this "intensive" lifestyle group was to lose at least 7 percent of body weight by eating less fat and increasing physical activity to 150 minutes or more per week. A second group in the study took metformin, a drug that is used to treat existing diabetes but is not yet approved for preventing the disease. A third group took a placebo, a pill with no active ingredients.

Those in the group that received intensive lifestyle-change training reduced their risk of developing type 2 diabetes by 58 percent. This strategy worked particularly well for participants age sixty and older, whose risk was reduced by 71 percent. Participants taking metformin reduced their risk by 31 percent, although this medication was less effective in people sixty and older. The results were so dramatic that the study was stopped one year earlier than planned so that this important information could be reported to the public. Results were published in the February 7, 2002, issue of the *New England Journal of Medicine*.

THE NURSES' HEALTH STUDY (NHS)

Another important study has surveyed approximately 250,000 women every two years for as long as thirty years. Although not a controlled, clinical trial, the Nurses' Health Study has provided an enormous amount of information on risk factors for major diseases in women. But results of such observational studies must be carefully interpreted. In these studies researchers observe, without benefit of control groups, how exposure to risk factors influences the likelihood of developing disease. They do not provide the definitive results of a clinical trial. For example, the NHS noted an association between estrogen use and decreased heart disease. We now know, through clinical trials, that estrogen actually *increases* the risk of heart disease.

Diabetes is one of the chronic diseases studied as part of the

NHS. Here is a sampling of the findings from the Nurses' Health Study that specifically concern type 2 diabetes in women:

➡ Being overweight or obese was the single most important predictor of type 2 diabetes; also associated with increased risk were lack of exercise and a diet low in cereal fiber and high in trans fats. Moderate alcohol consumption (one drink a day) was associated with a decrease in risk. If all these lifestyle factors were improved, the researchers calculated that the incidence of type 2 diabetes might be 90 percent lower.

➡ The amount of time spent watching television—a sedentary activity—was associated with an increased risk of obesity and type 2 diabetes. Even just walking around the house appeared to reduce risk, but brisk walking for one hour per day was associated with a greater risk reduction.

➡ Cigarette smoking was an important cause of certain cancers and heart disease, and may also be a risk factor for type 2 diabetes.

➡ In terms of reducing the risk of developing type 2 diabetes, walking seemed to be as effective as vigorous physical activity.

➡ Eating more nuts and peanut butter (in place of red meat, refined grain products like white bread, and processed meats like hot dogs) was associated with lower risk of type 2 diabetes.

➡ Women with long or very irregular menstrual cycles (usual length is twenty-six to thirty-one days)—which is associated with obesity and polycystic ovary syndrome (see Chapter 5)—had a significantly increased risk of developing type 2 diabetes. This risk was further increased by obesity.

PILLS TO PREVENT?

Several studies, including the DPP described above, have shown that medications currently being prescribed for diabetes or weight loss also appear to help prevent diabetes in those with prediabetes. None of them has as significant an effect as lifestyle changes and none at this point has been approved by the Federal Drug Administration (FDA) for the prevention of type 2 diabetes. It could well be that medications such as the metformin used in the Diabetes Prevention Program, when combined with lifestyle changes, will be even better at prevention.

That is not to say that you won't be taking pills. You may have to take medications to manage high blood pressure and cholesterol, if you aren't already. But here again, the same lifestyle changes that prevent diabetes are likely to help with blood pressure and cholesterol control as well.

If you're concerned about diabetes, the best advice is to lose weight, eat less fat and fewer calories, and get more physically active. Genes are not destiny with type 2 diabetes. Lifestyle risk factors can push your blood sugars up into diabetes. Taking action to modify such behaviors now can be the reset button that brings your levels down to normal.

WHY WEIGHT LOSS IS IMPORTANT

It is a simple fact that almost 70 percent of Americans are overweight. The rise in obesity in the United States has paralleled the rise in type 2 diabetes.

This is not just a coincidence. There are physiological reasons that these two epidemics are related and often go hand in hand. Obesity itself results in insulin resistance, a hallmark of prediabetes and a stepping-stone to type 2 diabetes. The body's cells resist the effect of insulin, so more insulin is required to maintain blood sugar levels. For every pound you gain, you increase your body's need for insulin. Diabetes develops when a person's ability to secrete insulin can't keep up with the rising demand for more insulin imposed by insulin resistance.

Most obese people have high levels of free fatty acids in their blood. Free fatty acids are a necessary source of fuel, but too high a level of them has been found to contribute to insulin resistance and perhaps to decreased insulin secretion from the pancreas. A high level of free fatty acids also triggers an inflammatory reaction that may lead to atherosclerosis, a narrowing of the blood vessels supplying the heart and brain that can result in heart attacks and stroke. Free fatty acids or other fat-cell products may in fact be a missing link—the reason obesity and type 2 diabetes can be a deadly combination and multiply the risk for heart disease.

The body's metabolism is most severely altered in those whose excess body fat is stored centrally around the abdomen, as opposed to around the hips and legs. This type of obesity is more typical in men than in women, although it becomes more common in women after menopause. A waist measurement of more than thirty-five inches is considered above normal in women.

The effect of these and other changes to body chemistry that occur with obesity—in concert with inherited factors—further deteriorates the fine-tuned feedback loops that keep the body producing the right amount of insulin.

An increasing number of people appear to have a cluster of metabolic disorders: obesity, insulin resistance, diabetes or prediabetes, high blood pressure, and abnormal lipids (cholesterols and triglycerides). Doctors refer to this group of conditions as metabolic syndrome. People diagnosed with metabolic syndrome appear to be at greater risk of developing cardiovascular disease, including heart attacks and stroke.

But the good news is that small weight losses can produce big health benefits. The Diabetes Prevention Program results show that a weight loss as low as 7 percent prevented diabetes and decreased blood glucose levels back toward the normal range. This amount of weight loss has also been linked to improvements in blood pressure and cholesterol levels, which are linked to heart disease and stroke. This is a case where we can perhaps turn back time.

THE MOTIVATION TO CHANGE

The results of the large clinical trials provide a game plan for how to prevent type 2 diabetes. We can share with you what worked in these studies, but to succeed you first have to believe in yourself. Ordinary women just like you have done it, and you can too. But you have to find your own reasons to follow the plan. It's not enough for us to tell you that it's good for you. You know that. Like actors who need to figure out what motivates the characters they are trying to play, you need to know what motivates you to make changes. You need to come up with reasons so compelling that they will get you through those stressful days when you'd like nothing better than to reach for a bag of chips.

We suggest that you start by making a list of the pros and cons of making changes to your diet and level of physical activity. Here are some examples:

Pros
I want to look in the mirror and feel better about myself.
I want to live a long life without the complications of diabetes.
I want to have children and live to see my grandchildren.
I want my children and the rest of my family to be healthy.

Cons
I'm depressed right now because a loved one just died or is very ill.
My family likes what I cook now.
I'm juggling a full-time job, child care, and household duties and have no time to exercise.
I've tried dieting and the weight always comes back.
I love to eat.

The diabetes prevention studies revealed the central importance of educating people on how to make lifestyle changes. The hurdles to success are your personal obstacles, the cons you've listed. But they are not insurmountable stone walls. With guidance, you can get over them.

The path to healthier living is gradual. Don't be frightened or discouraged about the amount of weight you need to lose. It might have taken you twenty or thirty years to become overweight, and it may take some time to lose the 7 percent we are recommending. The important thing is to head in the right direction and keep moving.

REWARD YOURSELF!

Set realistic goals and reward yourself as you reach them—a nonfood reward! Some examples: fresh flowers, a professional massage, a night out with just your girlfriends, money toward something you've been eyeing.

Your list of pros is your personal motivation to succeed. This is the list you tape to your refrigerator. It is what you go back to when you want to give up or after you lapse temporarily.

One way to look at change is as a marvelous opportunity. Here is a chance to lower your risk of developing diabetes, heart disease, and certain cancers, all the while feeling better about yourself. The cost of diabetes to society, in terms of medical expenditures and lost productivity, is estimated to be about $132 billion. The cost of a life not shortened or limited by complications of diabetes, priceless.

TIPPING THE SCALES

The key is to regain better balance in your life. The mantra is "calories in, calories out." To maintain a healthy weight, you should take in only as many calories as your body needs to function. If you take in more than you need—even a tiny bit more each day—your body stores the excess as fat and you gain weight. To lose weight, you must burn more calories than you consume. Physical activity helps tip the scales in this balancing act by burning more calories.

Losing weight is pretty easy. What's hard is keeping it off. Don't think in terms of going on a "diet," which implies something temporary. We're talking about starting a gradual process of introducing healthier habits into your life that will become part of who you are. That's why your personal plan for healthier living should start with foods you like to eat and activities you like to do. In this way you will not be depriving yourself; you will be making changes you can live with.

Although we know that changing your energy balance is critical—more calories "out" with activity than go "in" with food—the best path to achieving this goal is actively debated. There is conflicting evidence on the best route to weight loss, especially when the goal is to keep the weight off permanently and safely. That doesn't stop each new diet book from proclaiming that it has the unique and only scientific answer to how to lose weight best. Until very recently, however, we haven't had any reliable comparative data on which approach works best. What's becoming clearer is that the best approach may come down to finding a plan you can stick with. Most weight-loss programs fail simply because people don't stick with them.

IT'S NOT ONLY ABOUT THE FOOD ON YOUR PLATE . . .

- Remember that everyone has to eat, including you!
- You can become an "educated eater" by learning about different food groups, the truth about sugar substitutes, how to read food labels, and tradeoffs between foods you crave and foods that are healthy for you.
- Don't forget the effects of stress and emotional upheavals on your eating patterns.
- Realize that cravings during different points in your menstrual cycle can impact your eating.
- Strive for balance: intelligent decision-making about eating, combined with sensible exercise, matching your medication to what you eat, curbing your portion sizes, and modifying your caloric and fat intake.

Below are several popular approaches to weight loss. Remember, for any of them to work, you must take in fewer calories than you expend:

➡ low-carbohydrate/high-fat diets (Atkins and The South Beach Diet, for example)
➡ very low–fat/high complex-carbohydrate diets (the Pritikin and Ornish diets)
➡ commercial weight-loss programs, with a typical emphasis on lowering calories through special menus, portion control, and ongoing support (Weight Watchers, Jenny Craig, LA Weight Loss)

➡ low (800–1,400 calories per day) and very low (under 800) calorie diets, undertaken with medical supervision

➡ reduced-fat/50–60 percent carbohydrate diets, such as those advocated by the American Diabetes Association and used in the Diabetes Prevention Program; a variation is the Mediterranean diet (lots of grains, fruits, vegetables, olive oil, garlic, seafood, with meat and poultry in moderation)

WEIGHT-LOSS OPTIONS

Diet

Exercise

Medications:

   silbutramine (Meridia)

   orlistat (Xenical)

   phentermine

Surgery:

   vertical banded gastroplasty

   adjustable gastric banding

   Roux-en-Y gastric bypass

There is some question about the long-term safety of eating extremely low amounts of fat. High amounts of fats (as allowed in high-protein or low-carbohydrate diets) may increase insulin resistance, cholesterol levels, and weight gain in the long run. High-protein diets may also be bad for the kidneys and cause kidney stones. See Table 3.1 for a more detailed breakdown of the most popular approaches to weight loss.

INGREDIENTS FOR SUCCESS

Although we don't have the final answer to which approach works best, the studies that have achieved the most sustained weight loss

Table 3.1   Popular diet plans

Diet plan	Highlights
Very low fat	
Pritikin diet	Mostly vegetarian; combine with exercise; most successful in those newly diagnosed with diabetes
Ornish diet	Originally designed for prevention of heart disease; mostly vegetarian, higher in fiber and meant to be combined with exercise
Oslo diet	Includes increase in fish; tested in a nondiabetic population
Moderate fat	
Weight Watchers	Aim of all three plans is to reduce calories by 500–1,000 cal/
Jenny Craig	day without limiting nutrients
Nutri Systems	
Low carbohydrate/high fat	
Atkins	High protein/low carbohydrate/low fiber
Protein Power	High in saturated fat
Life without Bread	Low in fruits and vegetables
The Carbohydrate Addicts Diet	Low in fruits and vegetables
Other low carbohydrate	
The Zone Diet	Restricts simple sugars and refined carbohydrates
Sugar Busters	Allows fruits
South Beach	Emphasizes eating the "right" carbs
Reduced fat/50–60 percent carbohydrate	
American Diabetes Association	For all these plans, reduce fats, particularly saturated and trans
Mediterranean Diet	fats; eat a variety of fruits, vegetables, and whole grain carbs,
Diabetes Prevention Program	particularly those high in fiber; increase daily physical activity
American Heart Association	to burn calories

Source: Adapted from S. Cummings, J. Pratt, and L. Kaplan, "Evaluation and Management of Obesity," in *Primary Care of Women* (St. Louis: Mosby, 2002).

have restricted fat. Fat has the most calories of all the food groups. Exercise alone has only a small effect on weight loss, though it helps to lower blood sugars and keep weight off. We also know that another critical element to success is "self-monitoring," for example, keeping track of how much fat you consume and how much exercise you get on a daily basis.

The DPP demonstrated the importance of intensive counseling

about eating behaviors, checking in regularly on progress, and follow-up after weight-loss goals were reached. Participants were taught how to be "fat detectives," identifying the huge number of calories that are found in hidden fats they eat. They were shown how to shop for and cook healthier, low-fat versions of their favorite foods. They were also coached in identifying the factors in their current lifestyle that made it hard for them to eat more healthily and be more active. They were shown how to find solutions that worked for them.

Behavioral counseling also helped people overcome some of the most common hurdles to losing weight, such as negative thinking. In the past, you may have used one slip off a diet as an excuse to binge wildly. Next time, make your first meal after a slip a healthy one. You can break the cycle of binging by telling yourself that you are not a failure because of one slip. Positive thinking in this case would be: "I'm not a failure just because I overate at the party. Next time I'll have a healthy snack before I go to a party so I won't be tempted to eat high-fat foods out of hunger."

Although participants in the Diabetes Prevention Program kept track of their fat intake and physical activities on a daily basis for the first six months, the emphasis was not on counting calories. Some people, however, do seem to benefit from a more structured program that provides detailed menus they can follow.

Investigators from the DPP identified factors that were associated with success in reaching the 7 percent weight-loss goal. After six months of the study, the participants most likely to reach their weight-loss goal

➡ had greater dietary self-control than others;
➡ were more effective at achieving a low-fat diet; and
➡ did less frequent emotional eating (see below).

One year into the study, these determinants were still important indicators of success, as were lower levels of stress and less consumption of high-fat foods.

EAT FOR HUNGER, NOT EMOTIONS

One barrier to healthy eating is emotional eating, that is, eating not out of hunger but as a reaction to a situation or an emotion, such as sadness, boredom, loneliness, or stress. You can break this habit. The first step is to recognize if you are prone to emotional eating and then write down what triggers you to binge. For example, you might write: "I eat ice cream whenever I get into a fight with my husband/boyfriend/partner." Or, "I crave chocolate when I'm stressed out over work or about to get my period."

The second step is to think about things you can do instead of eating when these triggers occur. On your list of triggers, you might set a goal that next time you get into an argument, you will go for a walk and calmly think about what you want to say to your partner later, instead of eating ice cream. When work gets stressful, maybe you can suck on a sugarless candy instead of going to the vending machine for a candy bar.

Sometimes emotional eating has a physiological component. Some researchers have identified people they call "carbohydrate cravers." These people may eat normally at mealtimes, but in the late afternoon and evening they crave carbohydrate-rich snacks. Eating

---

SETTING GOALS

Some general principles that dietitians recommend in setting long-term lifestyle goals:

- Be realistic. Set reasonable goals you can reach and maintain.
- Reduce the calories you take in and increase the calories you burn.
- Increase activity levels gradually and by doing things you enjoy.
- Know that you can be fit no matter what your size.
- Be confident.
- Expect setbacks and don't be defeated by them. Look ahead, not back.
- Don't be embarrassed to ask for help.
- Be patient. There are no quick fixes.

---

carbohydrates may release a chemical messenger in the brain called serotonin, which regulates appetite as well as mood. Eating carbohydrates may be a form of self-medication for these people, who report feeling more relaxed and calm after eating them. For some women, carbohydrate craving may occur premenstrually.

We will deal with emotional eating, binge eating, and depression (which can also impede weight loss) in more detail in Chapter 6. But in general, identifying what makes you eat the wrong foods is a critical part of the formula for successful weight loss.

BUILD A BONFIRE FOR CALORIES

The "calories out" side of the formula for success is more straightforward than "calories in." Physical activity burns calories. To burn more calories than you have been, increase your physical activity. This includes increasing any body movement that expends energy—such as taking the stairs instead of an elevator, getting up to change channels rather than using the clicker, parking farther away from your destination. Even simple housework like vacuuming uses calories. But more calories are burned when the activity is brisk and sustained enough that it gets your heart pumping a little harder than usual. Various national guidelines recommend we do about thirty minutes of this "moderate" physical activity on most days of the week, but at least three times a week. Those who increase their physical activity are more likely to lose weight and keep the weight off.

A BALANCED DIET

Temptation is everywhere. High-fat, inexpensive foods are heavily advertised and widely available. Carbs and fats taste good. Although we need both for healthy living, they should be consumed in proper balance with other food groups. So what is a balanced diet?

The original food pyramid created by the U.S. Department of Agriculture

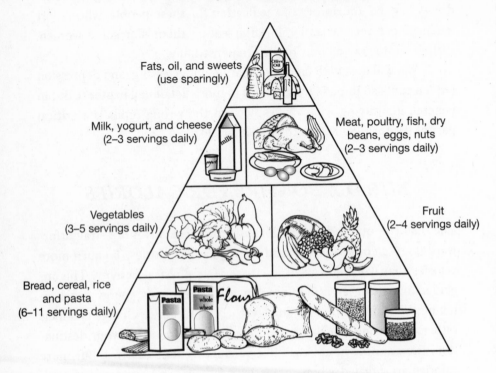

Fats, oil, and sweets (use sparingly)

Milk, yogurt, and cheese (2–3 servings daily)

Meat, poultry, fish, dry beans, eggs, nuts (2–3 servings daily)

Vegetables (3–5 servings daily)

Fruit (2–4 servings daily)

Bread, cereal, rice and pasta (6–11 servings daily)

The main elements of a balanced diet are proteins, carbohydrates, and fats. All three are essential for a healthy body to function. Most Americans consume more than enough of each of these nutrients. All three contain calories, but fat is the most fattening, not surprisingly. Fat contains more than twice the calories of the same amount of carbohydrates and proteins.

You can tinker with the amount and type of carbohydrates and proteins you eat—as myriad fad diets will direct—but the simplest way to lose weight is by eating less fat. In many instances, if you reduce your consumption of fats to recommended levels, you can naturally achieve a better balance among the other nutrients. The American Diabetes Association, the American Heart Association (AHA), and

An alternate food pyramid created by Dr. Walter C. Willett and the nutritional experts at the Harvard School of Public Health

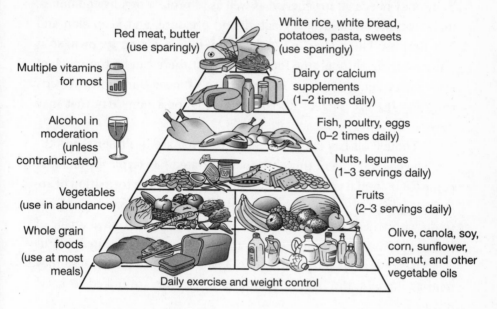

Red meat, butter (use sparingly)

White rice, white bread, potatoes, pasta, sweets (use sparingly)

Multiple vitamins for most

Dairy or calcium supplements (1–2 times daily)

Alcohol in moderation (unless contraindicated)

Fish, poultry, eggs (0–2 times daily)

Nuts, legumes (1–3 servings daily)

Vegetables (use in abundance)

Fruits (2–3 servings daily)

Whole grain foods (use at most meals)

Olive, canola, soy, corn, sunflower, peanut, and other vegetable oils

Daily exercise and weight control

The base of any healthy diet includes a variety of grains, fruits, and vegetables. The best advice available for preventing type 2 diabetes is to lose weight, eat less fat and fewer calories, and get more exercise.

various other government health agencies all recommend that no more than 30 percent of your daily calories come from fats.

The optimal balance of proteins and carbohydrates is more debatable. But we do know that a healthy diet contains carbohydrates in the form of whole grains, fruits, and vegetables. These foods contain fiber and other essential vitamins and minerals. Studies have indicated that fiber helps to control blood sugar and cholesterol levels. In Chapter 8 we will discuss carbohydrates in more detail.

> *The simplest way to lose weight is to eat less fat.*

Eating a variety of foods is key. If a diet plan is too restrictive, you won't stick with it for long.

NOT ALL FAT IS EQUAL

Your body needs fat for energy, as well as to protect organs and bones, make certain hormones, regulate blood pressure, and keep skin and hair healthy. The body can't make many fatty acids on its own, so it must get them through the food we eat. But there can be too much of even a good thing. If we eat more fat than we need—and most Americans do—the excess gets stored in fat cells for a rainy day that may never come. And so we get fatter.

Though all fats should be limited, some are healthier than others. The general rule of thumb is that saturated fats (typically fats that come from animal versus plant products) promote the formation of artery-clogging fatty deposits; unsaturated fats do not. "Saturation" has to do with whether the fatty acids contained in the fat have a pair of hydrogen atoms (saturated) or are missing them (unsaturated). Saturated fats and trans fatty acids are the worst types of fat because they tend to increase the blood cholesterol levels that are linked to heart disease.

We don't need to consume cholesterol. Our body makes all it needs in the liver. Although, as with fat, there are "good" (HDL) and "bad" (LDL) types of cholesterol in our bodies, there is no good type of cholesterol in the foods we eat.

Avoid saturated fats such as butter, shortening, fats on meats, bacon, and tropical oils like coconut and palm oil. These same foods are also high in cholesterol and promote high levels of LDL cholesterol in the bloodstream. Sour cream and cream cheese are saturated fats, but both come in lower-fat and nonfat versions.

Avoid trans fatty acids. Manufacturers created a new type of fat in an attempt to make unsaturated oils more stable and less likely to become rancid. Trans fatty acids can be found in margarines (stick versions have the most; tubs the least), baked goods (like packaged doughnuts, cookies, and cakes), snack foods (chips, crackers), fried foods, salad dressings, and any product that has an ingredient called "partially hydrogenated" or "hydrogenated" vegetable oil.

TYPES OF FATS

Trans fatty acids (avoid)	Saturated fats (eat small amounts)	Unsaturated fats (healthier options)
Packaged baked goods (cookies, doughnuts, crackers)	Bacon	*Monounsaturated:*
	Butter	Avocados
Chips (unless baked)	Meat fat and lard	Peanut butter
Mayonnaise (unless canola-based)	Tropical oils: coconut, palm	Nuts: almonds, peanuts, cashews
	Some creamy salad dressings	Oils: canola, olive
Deep-fried foods	Sour cream (low fat is ok)	*Polyunsaturated:*
Some margarines (tub or liquid form has less than harder, stick forms)	Cream cheese (low fat is ok)	Oils: corn, safflower, soybean
	Ice cream	Many salad dressings
	Chocolate	Fish (salmon, tuna)
		Margarine
		Mayonnaise (if canola oil–based)

Use "healthier" unsaturated fats—monounsaturated and polyunsaturated— in moderation. These fats have been shown to lower LDL cholesterol in the blood, although polyunsaturated fats may also lower HDL cholesterol. Monounsaturated fats are found in avocados, oils (olive, canola, peanut), peanut butter, and nuts (almonds, cashews, hazelnuts, peanuts). Polyunsaturated fats include certain oils (safflower, corn, soybean), high-fat fish such as salmon and tuna, and mayonnaise. Salmon is also high in omega-3 fats, which are heart-healthy.

KEEP A FOOD DIARY

One of the first steps toward a healthier diet is to record what you eat. We guarantee that you will be surprised by how much fat you are eating without knowing it. For a week or two, write down everything you drink and eat, including snacks, the cream and sugar in your coffee, and any sauces and dressings you might not think of separately as foods. Write down how the food is prepared (fried, boiled, broiled, grilled) and the size of the portions.

In the DPP, participants kept a food log and then were asked to circle which foods they thought were highest in fat. They continued to write down their daily fat intake for six months. Many studies have found that this sort of self-monitoring with food diaries is one of the most important criteria for successful weight loss.

Ideally, you too should consult with a dietitian about how best to reduce fat in your diet. A registered dietitian can help you develop a well-balanced eating plan tailored to your particular health concerns. It may well be that if you have a health condition—such as prediabetes, cardiovascular disease, or obesity—your health insurance will cover the cost of consultation with a dietitian. You may need a referral from your primary doctor or health care provider, who can also recommend local dietitians.

Whether or not you initially choose to see a dietitian, you should be aware of some general concepts essential to healthier living. In order to make positive lifestyle changes, you will need to learn to read food labels, develop low-fat strategies you can live with, and get moving to use up those fat stores.

Many people find it helpful to enlist a friend or partner to join them—someone to walk and talk with; someone to share low-fat recipes with. You might also get family members including children and grandchildren involved. But even if you don't, you may find that others will follow your lead when they see a lighter bounce in your step. With or without a partner, you *can* do this.

READING FOOD LABELS

There are three ways to eat less fat: eat smaller amounts of high-fat foods, eat high-fat foods less often, and eat lower-fat foods instead.

Sample nutrition label for
macaroni and cheese

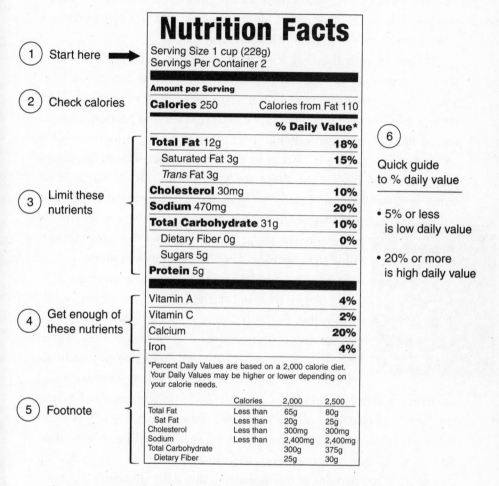

① Start here ➡

② Check calories

③ Limit these nutrients

④ Get enough of these nutrients

⑤ Footnote

⑥ Quick guide to % daily value

Nutrition Facts

Serving Size 1 cup (228g)
Servings Per Container 2

Amount per Serving

Calories 250   Calories from Fat 110

	% Daily Value*
Total Fat 12g	**18%**
Saturated Fat 3g	**15%**
Trans Fat 3g	
Cholesterol 30mg	**10%**
Sodium 470mg	**20%**
Total Carbohydrate 31g	**10%**
Dietary Fiber 0g	**0%**
Sugars 5g	
Protein 5g	

Vitamin A	**4%**
Vitamin C	**2%**
Calcium	**20%**
Iron	**4%**

*Percent Daily Values are based on a 2,000 calorie diet. Your Daily Values may be higher or lower depending on your calorie needs.

	Calories	2,000	2,500
Total Fat	Less than	65g	80g
Sat Fat	Less than	20g	25g
Cholesterol	Less than	300mg	300mg
Sodium	Less than	2,400mg	2,400mg
Total Carbohydrate		300g	375g
Dietary Fiber		25g	30g

• 5% or less is low daily value

• 20% or more is high daily value

A first step to weight loss is to be able to identify the amount and type of fat, and the number of calories in a food product. (Food and Drug Administration.)

The first step is to be able to identify how much fat and how many calories from fat are in a given food you purchase at the store. It may take some time at first to read every packaged food label, but soon you will learn what to buy and what to avoid.

Remember that our strategy here is not just to count calories but to cut out extra calories that you've been eating in fats. If you concentrate on healthier eating—more whole grain products, vegetables and fruits, skim instead of whole or 2 percent milk—you'll naturally reduce calories without having to count up the calorie content of everything you eat. Add more physical activity to the mix, and you may find that's all you have to do to gradually lose weight.

So it's worth the time it takes to read the Nutrition Facts label that is now required on most packaged foods. At the top of the label you'll see the serving size and number of servings per container. Take note of this because if you eat more than that serving portion, the values of fat, calories, and other nutrients listed will also increase. One serving of macaroni and cheese in the sample label shown, for example, is one cup. In that cup there are 250 calories, 110 of which come from "bad" saturated and trans fat. Keep in mind that the average overweight woman (about 180 pounds) who is physically inactive burns about 2,000 calories a day. Use this as a guide to determine if you're using up too much of your daily allotment of fat and calories in one serving.

Generally speaking, if you cut back your usual calories by about 400 per day, you can lose roughly a pound every ten days.

Notice that on the right side of the label is a column called "% Daily Value." This tells you how much one serving of the product contributes to what nutrition experts have determined should be our daily allowance of the nutrients listed. These figures are based on an average daily intake of 2,000 calories. So on our sample label, the total fat in one serving of macaroni and cheese represents 18 percent of the daily recommended amount of fat that should be in your diet. For a healthy diet, you want your total intake of fat in a day to add up to less than 100 percent of the recommended daily allowance.

Your total daily intake of saturated fat should also add up to less than 100 percent, as should your daily intake of cholesterol. Government agencies have not yet established a daily value for trans fats, so none is listed, nor is a percentage indicated for sugar or protein.

One confusing issue to sort out when shopping is the difference between claims of "fat free" versus "low fat" versus "reduced fat." The federal government has established these criteria:

→ fat free: less than one-half gram of fat per serving

→ low fat: 3 grams or less of fat per serving

→ reduced fat or less fat: at least 25 percent less fat than the regular version

Reducing portion sizes is also important. "Supersizing"—providing more food for less money—is a technique that has reaped profits

Reduced-fat vs. nonfat milk

Reduced-fat milk
2% milkfat

Nonfat milk

Nutrition Facts

Serving Size 1 cup (236ml)
Servings Per Container 1

Amount per Serving

Calories 120	Calories from Fat 45
	% Daily Value*
Total Fat 5g	**8%**
Saturated Fat 3g	**15%**
Trans Fat 0g	
Cholesterol 20mg	**7%**
Sodium 120mg	**5%**
Total Carbohydrate 11g	**4%**
Dietary Fiber 0g	**0%**
Sugars 11g	
Protein 9g	**17%**

Vitamin A 10% • Vitamin C 4%
Calcium 30% • Iron 0% • Vitamin D 25%

*Percent Daily Values are based on a 2,000 calorie diet. Your Daily Values may be higher or lower depending on your calorie needs.

Nutrition Facts

Serving Size 1 cup (236ml)
Servings Per Container 1

Amount per Serving

Calories 80	Calories from Fat 0
	% Daily Value*
Total Fat 0g	**0%**
Saturated Fat 0g	**0%**
Trans Fat 0g	
Cholesterol Less than 5mg	**0%**
Sodium 120mg	**5%**
Total Carbohydrate 11g	**4%**
Dietary Fiber 0g	**0%**
Sugars 11g	
Protein 9g	**17%**

Vitamin A 10% • Vitamin C 4%
Calcium 30% • Iron 0% • Vitamin D 25%

*Percent Daily Values are based on a 2,000 calorie diet. Your Daily Values may be higher or lower depending on your calorie needs.

Note the significant difference in calories and fat between the reduced-fat (2 percent) milk and the nonfat milk. Nonfat milk has 80 calories, none of which comes from fat. Reduced-fat milk, by contrast, has 120 calories, 45 (or more than one-third) of which come from fat. Both are equally good sources of calcium, which women need for strong bones.

for food companies but has led to overeating and obesity among Americans. The size of individual muffins, candy bars, and soft drinks, for example, has grown over the past few decades, as have portion sizes served at restaurants (the National Heart, Lung, and Blood Institute refers to this phenomenon as "portion distortion"). Bigger portions mean we take in more calories.

In many cases we end up eating the equivalent of two serving sizes instead of one. When you first start thinking about portion sizes, you may want to get out the measuring cup or spoons. Table 3.2 gives you an idea of how to eyeball portion sizes for those times when it's not practical to measure or weigh your food.

LABEL LINGO

Free: No amount of, or a trivial amount of, one or more of these components: fat, saturated fat, cholesterol, sodium, sugars, and calories

Low fat: 3 g. or less per serving

Low saturated fat: 1 g. or less per serving

Low sodium: 140 mg. or less per serving

Very low sodium: 35 mg. or less per serving

Low cholesterol: 20 mg. or less and 2 g. or less of saturated fat per serving

Low calorie: 40 calories or less per serving

Lean: Less than 10 g. fat; 4.5 g. or less of saturated fat; less than 95 mg. cholesterol per serving and per 100 g.

Extra lean: Less than 5 g. fat; less than 2 g. of saturated fat; less than 95 mg. cholesterol per serving and per 100 g.

High: Contains 20 percent or more of the Daily Value for a particular nutrient in a serving

Good source: Contains 10–19 percent of the Daily Value for a particular nutrient in a serving

Reduced: At least 25 percent less of a nutrient or of calories than the regular, or reference, product

Note: mg = milligrams; g = grams
Source: "The Food Label," FDA (www.cfsan.fda.gov/~dms/fdnewlab.html).

Table 3.2   Translating portion sizes

.5 cup of rice or pasta	= size of an ice-cream scoop
1 cup of salad greens	= size of a baseball
.5 cup of chopped fruit or vegetables	= size of a lightbulb
1.5 ounces of cheese	= size of four dice
3 ounces of meat or fish	= size of a deck of cards
2 tablespoons of peanut butter	= size of a ping pong ball
1 teaspoon of oil	= size of your thumb tip

Source: "Better Health and You," National Institute of Diabetes, Digestive, and Kidney Disease (http://win.niddk.nih.gov/publications/better_health.htm).

MODIFYING A RECIPE

Often we don't even realize how much fat something has because it is hidden. You can see and cut off excess fats that cover red meats, chicken, and pork. We know deep-fried foods like french fries and fried chicken have a lot of fat and should be kept to special occasions. But the fat marbled in red meats and contained in sauces, batters, and baked products is less obvious unless we look at the ingredients. It is well worth the extra time to bake and prepare meals from scratch so that you have control over the ingredients.

You can find low-fat versions of your favorite recipes or make lower-fat substitutions. Your family may initially resist changing a much-loved dish, but they will often adapt if you find a tasty variation of it. Say your husband has loved pork chops smothered in stuffing since his childhood. Why not make the dish with thinner chops and smother it with sautéed onions and mushrooms instead of stuffing? Keep a file of the lower-fat recipes that you and your family enjoy most. These can then become your new favorites.

Ohio State University's Human Nutrition and Food Management program suggests the following recipe substitutions for a low-fat diet:

➡ To reduce fat in baked products, use less oil. For example, if a cookie or muffin recipe calls for 1 cup of oil, use 2/3 of a cup instead. (Do not reduce oil for yeast breads or pie crusts.)

➡ Instead of using solid fats such as shortening, lard, and butter, use vegetable oil (corn, canola, or peanut oil). When making this exchange, use about 1/4 less, so if a recipe calls for 1/4 cup butter (4 tablespoons), use 3 tablespoons of oil instead.

➡ In baking, replace sour cream with the same amount of plain low-fat or nonfat yogurt, or with buttermilk or low-fat cottage cheese.

➡ Use skim milk or 1 percent milk instead of whole milk or half-and-half. Evaporated skim milk has extra richness.

➡ Reduce sugar by 1/4 to 1/3 in baked goods and desserts, and substitute the amount that was omitted with flour. If a recipe calls for 1 cup of sugar, try 3/4 cup sugar and 1/4 cup flour, for example. (This substitution will not work for yeast breads.)

OTHER STRATEGIES TO REDUCE FAT

Women need calcium and other nutrients to prevent osteoporosis, a weakening of the bones that can lead to a hunched back and fractures. So foods with calcium—milk, cheese, yogurt, and dark-green vegetables, for example—are essential. Milk is an easy way to get calcium, but it is also high in fat unless you drink skim or 1 percent.

To reduce fat further, bake, broil, steam, roast, or grill your food instead of frying it. Sauté foods with vegetable oils instead of butter. Add herbs and spices instead of sauces for high flavor and low fat. Trim the fat from meats and remove the skin from chicken.

If you are accustomed to cleaning your plate, use a smaller plate with smaller portions. A reasonable portion of meat, for example, is the size of a deck of cards or a hamburger bun.

If you snack between meals, choose healthier treats like carrot sticks, celery stuffed with peanut butter, rice cakes, almonds, unflavored yogurt, air-popped or microwave popcorn (without oil or butter), pretzels, and of course fruit. Try stoneground corn chips with guacamole instead of potato chips and onion dip. Instead of eating right out of a box, pour a reasonable amount in a bowl and put the rest away.

HEALTHY SNACKS

(less than 15 grams of carbohydrate* and 5 grams of fat)

1 cup of raw vegetables

1/2 apple

1 small fruit

1/2 cup applesauce

3 cups of air-popped popcorn

8 saltine crackers

1 "lite" low-fat yogurt or cottage cheese

*15 grams of carbohydrate = 1 serving

Restaurants often have low-fat items on the menu, or you can always request that your choice be broiled, for example, instead of fried. (See Chapter 8 for more tips on eating out.) Even if you decide to splurge on a special occasion, share your entrée or dessert. Consider alternatives to high-fat desserts, such as a baked apple, a bowl of berries, or fruit crisps; ginger snaps, vanilla wafers, and oatmeal cookies; angel food cake; jelly beans or hard candy; and fruit popsicles. (See Table 3.3 for a list of articifial sweeteners, some of which you can bake and cook with.)

Remember, too, that just because something is labeled low fat or nonfat doesn't mean you can eat unlimited quantities of it. These foods can still add up to a lot of calories.

All this talk about change may well be making you anxious. Right about now, you may feel like reaching for a cookie or a bowl of ice cream. Well, maybe this one last time. But remember the saying: Tomorrow is the first day of the rest of your life. Anxiety doesn't have to make you eat junk food. It can make you eat healthily if you establish a new habit.

This doesn't mean you can't occasionally indulge in a high-fat treat. The operative word is *occasionally*. Have those barbecued ribs

Table 3.3 Sugar-free and artificial sweeteners

Chemical name	Brand name	Sweetness compared with sugar (applies to all sweeteners in class)	Can be used for hot foods	Can be used for cold foods
Acesultame-potassium	DiabetiSweet Sweet One	200 times sweeter	Yes	Yes
Aspartame*	Equal Nutrasweet Sweetmate	160–220 times sweeter	Yes, but if baking, only if cooked for <20 minutes	Yes
Saccharin**	Sucaryl Sugar Twin Sweet n' Low Sweet Magic Zero cal	200–700 times sweeter	Yes	Yes
Sucralose	Splenda	400–800 times sweeter	Yes	Yes

* Not for use by those with phenylketonuria (PKU).
** Not safe in pregnancy.
Note: Stevia, an herbal sweetener not approved for use by the FDA in the United States, is sold as a "dietary supplement" by some health food stores.
Source: Adapted from www.diabetes123.com.

once in a while—just fill the plate with veggies and greens, too. The main thing is to choose what you eat wisely. Keep track of the fats. Enjoy your food.

KEEP MOVING

The other side of the calories in/calories out formula is calories out. You need to burn more calories than you take in so that your body uses some of its fat stores for energy. You do this by increasing your activity level.

Participants in the Diabetes Prevention Program were encouraged to begin eating more healthily for a few weeks before introducing more physical activity into their lives. Some people, though, chose to start by increasing physical activity first. It's up to you. The main thing is not to make too many changes at once.

If national statistics are any indication, we can pretty much bet that most of you reading this are not physically active enough. Forty percent of Americans report no leisure-time physical activity, and many of our jobs are entirely sedentary. Still, everyone has her own individual starting point. As with adopting healthier eating habits, one way to begin is by listing everything you do over the next few days that gets you breathing a little heavily. For some, just getting out of a chair is hard work. This counts too. The list is for your eyes only. Keep it to look back on in six months to a year. If you gradually increase your activities, you'll be amazed at how far you can come.

It's a good idea to see your health care provider before increasing your physical exertion to make certain that doing so is safe for you. This is especially important if you have heart disease, are obese (a body mass index of 30 or greater), are over fifty, or have back or knee problems. Just remember, you can be fit and active no matter what size or shape your body is in.

There are essentially four approaches to leading a more active life:

→ Move more in everyday life: walk while talking on a remote phone, get up to change the channels on the television, park farther away from the store, walk down the hall to tell someone something at the office rather than calling or emailing, do housework, garden.
→ Do aerobic exercise: walk briskly three to five times a week, take aerobic dance or step classes, jog, swim, bicycle, dance for most of an evening.
→ Strength train: lift weights or do progressive weight training, do push-ups and sit-ups.
→ Practice mind and body exercises: do yoga, pilates, or tai chi.

Ideally, we should all exercise at least thirty minutes on most days of the week. It doesn't even have to be in one session each day; for example, you could do three ten-minute sessions daily. In the DPP, participants worked up to and exceeded the goal of 150 minutes per week of moderate-intensity physical activity (activities that make you

Table 3.4 Get physical: types of exercise

Exercise	Examples	How it helps
Endurance	Brisk walking Bike riding Dancing Stair climbing Gardening	Increases heart rate and improves blood flow through heart and lungs
Strength or resistance	Weight lifting Weight pushing Resistance band stretching Fitness machines (Nautilus, Stair-Master, treadmill)	Tones muscles; builds new muscle; strengthens spine; builds upper body, which prevents osteoporosis
Stretching	Side hip rotation Touching your toes	Improves flexibility and freedom of movement
Balance	Side leg raising Standing on one foot for as long as you can	Decreases risk of falls, especially for the elderly

Source: Bruce Agnew, *Diabetes Forecast* (March 2005), p. 52 (American Diabetes Association).

breathe harder than usual; see Table 3.4). Although most people chose walking, the possibilities are endless. Here are just a few:

- ➡ brisk walking, hiking
- ➡ dancing (Latin, line, aerobic)
- ➡ swimming or water exercise (laps, water aerobics, or exercise classes)
- ➡ skating
- ➡ rowing (canoe, kayak)
- ➡ tennis
- ➡ jump roping (for at least ten minutes with breaks)
- ➡ karate, kickboxing, or other martial arts
- ➡ gardening, raking leaves
- ➡ sex (burns as many calories as walking!)

The important thing is to find something you like and stick with it. As you become more fit and confident (and you will), you might vary your routine by trying other activities.

If you haven't been active to this point, it is important to build up to your goal gradually over several months. Walking is an easy way to start because all you need are good shoes and a safe route. You might start the first week or two by walking slowly for five minutes, followed by brisker walking for two to five minutes, and then walking slowly again to cool down. Even a total time of ten minutes is a good start. Set your own goals based on how you feel as you're moving. Don't rush to add more minutes, but don't be too easy on yourself either. But by all means stop if you experience any chest pain. Women who already have diabetes, particularly those with neuropathy (more on that next chapter), need to wear properly fitted shoes and regularly inspect their feet for blisters or sores.

NO MATTER WHAT YOUR SHAPE OR SIZE

We recognize that very large women have special challenges to becoming more active. They might be self-conscious around other people, need specially sized equipment, or have joint problems that make it difficult to do weight-bearing exercise. The National Institute of Diabetes and Digestive and Kidney Disease, through its Weight-Control Information Network, publishes an excellent booklet called "Active at Any Size." It has many suggestions for safe activities and resources (books, videos, websites, clothing, and organizations) for larger women. You can call the Weight-Control Information Network toll-free at 1-877-946-4627 or view the information online at www.niddk.nih.gov and search for "active at any size."

Various other government agencies, such as the Centers for Disease Control, the Food and Drug Administration's Office of Women's Health, and the Department of Health and Human Services' National Women's Health Information Center (4woman.gov) also have online programs geared to women who want to eat sensibly and be more active. The American Heart Association and the American Diabetes Association can help, too. Many women have successfully turned to national commercial programs such as Weight Watchers and Curves to help them adopt a healthier lifestyle.

Most women find that though they initially dread exercise, they eventually begin to look forward to it. In addition to improving your health, physical activity will make you look and feel better, sleep better, and have more energy. It's a way to relieve stress. Your mood will improve. You may meet new friends. And what's good for you will be good for your family, too.

PREVENTING TYPE 2 DIABETES IN CHILDREN

It is estimated that one out of three children born in the year 2000 will develop diabetes in her lifetime—a figure that government officials calculate will increase even more dramatically in the coming years if something is not done. This should be an added incentive for you to eat more healthfully and live a more active lifestyle. You will benefit not only yourself but also your children and grandchildren, those you have now and those to come.

If you are at risk for developing type 2 diabetes, it is very possible that your children or future children will also be at risk. They share your genes as well as your home environment. (See Chapter 5 for a discussion of genetic predisposition to diabetes.) Children and teenagers at greatest risk are those who are overweight or obese and have a family history of the disease.

In the past, type 2 diabetes was considered an adult disease. But not anymore. This is especially alarming since the younger children are when they get the disease, the longer they live with it, and the greater the risks of life-threatening complications.

Remember, the same strategies for preventing type 2 diabetes apply to children as well as to adults: control weight, eat more healthfully, and be physically active. Here are some specific tips to help the children in your life prevent diabetes:

➡ Devote at least one day a week to a physical activity in which the whole family participates.

➡ Go for walks or bike rides together. Encourage team sports or active video games such as Dance Dance Revolution, where players follow arrows and move their feet to the beat of popular songs.

➡ Limit television, computer, and video games to an agreed-upon limit per day, such as no more than two hours.

➡ Drink water and low-fat milk instead of soda, sports drinks, and juice.

➡ Limit fast food and unhealthy snacks. Reduce portion sizes at home.

➡ Serve fruits and vegetables at each meal.

➡ Don't use food as a reward or eat while watching television.

➡ Think of positive, nonfood rewards for children who accomplish activity and healthy-eating goals.

The best thing you can do for your overweight children or grandchildren is give them the opportunity to live a healthier life. Your best chance at success in this regard is to involve the whole family in adopting healthier habits. Everyone will benefit from low-fat meals and family activity. Remember, exercise does not have to be unpleasant—grab the family and go for a hike or a brisk walk around the neighborhood, clean up the yard, or dance to your favorite music. The possibilities, like the rewards, are endless.

4

Medical Complications

For months Barbara, a forty-five-year-old marketing executive, had been experiencing fatigue and irritability, which she attributed to a stressful job. She was also losing weight despite eating more, and had chronic vaginal and yeast infections, which she had never had before. She was tested for diabetes and was surprised to learn that the reason she was feeling so bad was that, at 500, her blood sugar was very high. She started taking insulin and began to feel better almost immediately. Her doctor recommended an eye examination, which did not reveal any problems.

For those of you who already have diabetes or prediabetes, the potential medical complications may understandably loom large. Diabetes can affect the normal functioning of many other parts of the body besides the pancreas, such as the eyes, kidneys, nerves, and circulatory system, which carries blood to the heart, brain, and limbs. These complications are literally a threat to life and limb whether you have type 1 or type 2 diabetes. But we have convincing evidence that you can take steps to prevent or at least delay each of these potential health problems.

Complications may seem like ticking time bombs, but they can be defused. First you must know what you are up against. In this chapter we talk about some of the most common complications of diabetes. Though they can be frightening, they are by no means your fate. But quite frankly, you do have to take action—or one or more of these complications could be in your future.

Some complications are more prevalent in those with type 1 diabetes than in those with type 2, and vice versa. But clearly everyone with diabetes is at risk of developing one or more complications over time. The simple fact is that over a long period of time, high blood glucose levels can damage the blood vessels and other parts of the eyes, the kidneys, and the nervous system. High blood pressure and abnormal cholesterol levels compound these problems. If you have type 1 or type 2 diabetes, you must see your health care providers regularly— even if you feel fine—so they can screen you for these complications and their risk factors.

KNOWLEDGE IS POWER

Surveys have shown that most people with diabetes are not aware of the extent to which the disease puts them at risk for serious health problems, particularly heart disease and stroke. Women may not know that the protective effect of hormones that usually reduces their risk of heart disease before menopause is seemingly erased by diabetes. Heart disease is the number one cause of death for women with diabetes. Whereas deaths from heart disease in general have been declining in the United States, even among diabetic men, such deaths are rising among women with diabetes.

Research has shown several ways that people can significantly reduce their risk of coronary heart disease and other complications of

PREVENTING CORONARY HEART DISEASE

Heart disease is the number one cause of death for women with diabetes, but you can prevent it. Here's how:

• Increase daily exercise and maintain an ideal body weight.

• Lower cholesterol and fat in your diet.

• Quit smoking.

• Follow your doctor's recommendations, which might include:

> *Tests*
> –Fasting cholesterol panel
> –EKG (electrocardiogram)
> –Exercise stress test or echocardiography
>
> *Medication*
> –Cholesterol-lowering medication (statins are often the first-line medications)
> –Blood pressure–lowering medication (ACE inhibitors or beta blockers are often first choices; thiazide diuretics may also be used)
> –Aspirin daily
> –Pills or insulin to achieve lower blood sugar and more intensive diabetes control

diabetes. These include careful, "tight" control of blood glucose, blood pressure, and lipids (such as cholesterol levels); and taking aspirin to prevent heart disease.

The vascular system of the body includes the blood vessels—the arteries, veins, and capillaries—that move blood around the body. Microvascular (or small blood vessel) complications, such as damage to the eyes, kidneys, and nerves, are the major risk for young people with type 1 diabetes, although they are also at increased risk for macrovascular (or large blood vessel) problems as they get older. Heart disease and other macrovascular complications are the leading cause of death and disability for both women and men with type 2 diabetes. But people with type 2 diabetes are also prone to microvascular complica-

Complications of diabetes

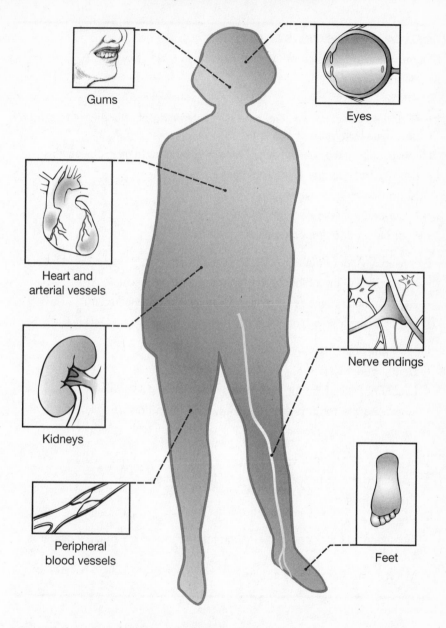

Whether you have type 1 or type 2 diabetes, problems can develop in many organs of the body. Over a long period of time, high blood sugar levels can damage blood vessels—a problem made worse by high blood pressure and abnormal cholesterol levels—and nerves. These complications are *not* inevitable.

MEDICAL COMPLICATIONS OF DIABETES

Macrovascular (large blood vessel) diseases:

- Heart disease
- Stroke
- Peripheral vascular disease, narrowing/stiffening of arteries in the extremities, usually in the feet and legs

Microvascular (small blood vessel) and neuropathic (nerve) diseases:

- Diabetic retinopathy (eye problems)
- Nephropathy (kidney disease)
- Neuropathy (nerve damage)
- Foot ulcers and amputation

Emergency ("acute metabolic") complications:

- Ketoacidosis (high blood sugar and ketones in blood)
- Hyperosmolar coma (very high blood sugar and dehydration)
- Hypoglycemia (low blood sugar)

Other complications:

- Dental gum disease
- Infections: skin, bladder, and others
- Increased risk for depression, anxiety, and eating disorders
- Carpal tunnel syndrome

Complications during pregnancy:

- Increased risk of miscarriage, if poorly controlled
- Preeclampsia
- Premature labor
- Increased risk for congenital malformations (not in gestational diabetes mellitus)
- Macrosomia (large baby at birth)

tions; many already show early signs of eye, kidney, and nerve problems by the time they are diagnosed.

We refer to macrovascular and microvascular complications as "long-term" because they usually require many years to develop. "Acute metabolic" complications, which we'll cover at the end of the chapter, signal that the body is in crisis and you must get medical help right away.

TAKING CONTROL

The most important thing you can do to reduce the development and progression of diabetes complications is to control blood glucose levels, blood pressure, and lipid levels (including LDL and HDL cholesterols and triglycerides). We now have evidence that the greatest benefits are probably achieved when you manage to control all three levels at the same time. You will also need to stick with a diet and activity plan. Almost all people with diabetes will benefit by following these strategies.

Each of you with diagnosed diabetes starts with your own palette of risks. You may already know from tests done after diagnosis, for example, that you have early signs of eye disease. Maybe heart disease runs in your family. As we detail each of the potential complications later in this chapter, we will provide specific strategies that are known to help prevent or slow each of them.

TIGHT GLUCOSE CONTROL

Control of blood sugar is the summit of the mountain, the goal to strive for and keep striving for. Remember, depending on the type of diabetes you have, your body either makes no insulin or does not make enough to meet your needs. This means that insulin is not able to do its job of getting glucose and other nutrients into the cells of the body, where they provide energy and help promote growth and development.

Somehow you need to make up for this absolute (type 1) or relative (type 2) lack of insulin. Discoveries and innovations in the past century have made this possible.

The goal of diabetes therapy is to help you maintain glucose levels as close to the nondiabetic range as is safely possible throughout the day—before and after meals, when you are awake, when you are asleep, during menstruation, and during special circumstances such as illness and stress. A healthy pancreas measures glucose levels constantly and secretes the right amount of insulin to keep glucose levels in a very tight range. Depending on the type of diabetes you have, you can achieve near-normal glucose levels by adjusting diet, exercise, and insulin or other glucose-lowering medications. Self-monitoring of blood glucose—which we describe in Chapter 7—often plays an important role in diabetes therapy.

For those with type 1 diabetes, tight or intensive control of glucose is accomplished by checking glucose levels and adjusting insulin doses—given by injection three or more times a day or delivered continuously through an insulin pump—based on your glucose levels, diet, and other factors. Standard glucose control in the past consisted of measuring urine or blood glucose and injecting insulin once or twice daily. But the results of a large clinical trial reported in 1993 showed definitively that the intensive approach could reduce the development of retinopathy by 76 percent and, in those who already had some evi-

---

GLUCOSE CONTROL TARGETS OUTSIDE OF PREGNANCY

Blood glucose (daily testing through self-monitoring):

Before meals: should be 80–120 mg/dl

One to two hours after meals: should be less than 180 mg/dl

Before bed: 100–140 mg/dl

Hemoglobin A_{1c} (HgbA$_{1c}$): Aim for as close to the nondiabetic range as possible (4–6.1 percent), and certainly less than 7 percent. Generally, your overall glucose control will be confirmed every three to four months with an HgbA$_{1c}$ in your doctor's office.

---

dence of eye disease, could slow the progression by 54 percent. The Diabetes Control and Complications Trial (DCCT), as the study was called, also showed that intensive therapy could reduce the development of kidney disease by 39 percent and further progression of the disease by 54 percent. Neuropathy (nerve disease) was reduced by 60 percent.

The goal in the DCCT, which should be your personal goal as well, was to keep the HgbA$_{1c}$ (glycohemoglobin) level at or below 7 percent. The HgbA$_{1c}$ test reflects the average glucose levels over the previous two to three months. Pre-meal glucose levels should be between 80 and 120 mg/dl, and the peak levels two hours after meals should be less than 180.

Tight control is not easy. In the United States, the average HgbA$_{1c}$ for people with diabetes is about 8 percent, even though lower HgbA$_{1c}$ is clearly better. In the DCCT, lower HgbA$_{1c}$ was associated with a dramatic decrease in the risk of complications. For example, for every 10 percent reduction in HgbA$_{1c}$—going from 10 to 9 percent or from 8 to 7.2, the risk of developing retinopathy was reduced by about 43 percent.

> For each 10 percent reduction in blood glucose levels, you reduce your rate of certain complications by 43 percent.

The long-term follow-up study of the DCCT has shown that intensive therapy has enduring benefits. Even though, on average, the HgbA$_{1c}$ levels of the original intensive-therapy participants has risen over time from 7.2 percent to almost 8 percent, they remained better off than those in the original study who had followed the less-intensive approach. The most recent results from the long-term follow-up have shown that intensive therapy decreased the rate of cardiovascular disease by 42 percent.

Intensive control is effective in slowing progression of established complications, but it is even more powerful in preventing the development of new complications. We now think that it is extremely important to practice intensive glucose control as early in the disease process as possible, before signs of problems develop.

People with type 2 diabetes also benefit from intensive glucose control. In 1998, the largest and longest clinical trial of type 2 diabetes—the United Kingdom Prospective Diabetes Study (UKPDS)—confirmed this fact after following men and women with type 2 diabetes for as long as twenty years. They found that changes in diet alone did not control glucose levels over time and did not prevent or delay microvascular complications as well as intensive treatment with glucose-lowering medications. Less clear in this study was the usefulness of tight blood sugar control for decreasing the occurrence of macrovascular complications. The UKPDS did find, however, that controlling high blood pressure helped prevent both micro- and macrovascular complications.

We know that people with either type 1 or type 2 diabetes benefit from lowering their glucose levels to as near normal as possible. In type 1 diabetes and in insulin-treated type 2 diabetes, accomplishing this goal requires "self-monitoring," measuring the level of glucose in the blood and responding accordingly. In Chapter 7 we will discuss more specifically how to achieve this goal whether you have type 1 or type 2 diabetes.

Women may have an even more difficult time than men keeping glucose levels stable because blood sugar levels fluctuate during the menstrual cycle, during pregnancy, and after menopause. But women who practice intensive control of their blood glucose say that they feel better. They have more energy; they don't have that "washed-out" feeling, increased thirst and urination, or the frequent bladder and vaginal infections that come when blood sugars are too high. And as a bonus, they have a substantially reduced risk of developing the eye, kidney, and nerve complications that can otherwise severely impair their health.

BLOOD PRESSURE CONTROL

High blood pressure (hypertension) is extremely common in people with diabetes, especially type 2 diabetes. Treating hypertension aggressively through drug therapy and diet can reduce the possibility of heart disease and stroke by more than 25 percent and microvascular eye and kidney complications by about 33 percent. If left untreated, however, the combination of diabetes and hypertension more than doubles the likelihood of heart disease or stroke.

Currently, hypertension is somewhat arbitrarily defined as a blood pressure of 140/90 mmHg or greater. Blood pressure is the pressure that blood puts on the walls of the blood vessels as it travels around the body. It's like water going through a hose. Pressure should be high enough to allow blood to reach all cells in the body, but not so high that it strains the walls of the vessels. Temporary surges in blood pressure occur when we are excited or stressed, but continuous strain on the blood vessel walls over time silently damages the vessels and the organs fed by those vessels, such as the brain, heart, kidney, and eyes. Hypertension is called a silent killer because the vast majority of people affected have no symptoms.

If you have diabetes, your goals for blood pressure control are even more strict than for nondiabetics. The first number (systolic blood pressure, the pressure when the heart contracts) should be less than 130, and the second number (diastolic blood pressure, the pressure at the moment the heart relaxes) less than 80. For people with kidney disease, blood pressure goals are even more strict.

Depending on how high your blood pressure is, your physician may start by recommending lifestyle changes: less salt, weight loss, increased physical activity, and giving up cigarettes if you smoke. All these strategies have been shown to reduce blood pressure. If the reduction is not enough to reach the desired blood pressure, drug treatment will be added (see Table 4.1). A drug called an ACE (angiotensin-converting enzyme) inhibitor is often the first medicine tried to reduce high blood pressure for someone with diabetes. But depending on your risk profile, you might be prescribed an ARB (angiotensin receptor blocker), a beta blocker, and/or a diuretic. Often it takes two or more medicines to reach the targeted blood pressure.

In some instances, hypertension medicine is prescribed even if

Table 4.1   Common medications to lower blood pressure

Women with diabetes need to lower their blood pressure below 130/80 mmHg. This can be accomplished through diet, weight loss, increased physical activity, and quitting smoking. If these measures don't work, your doctor will prescribe one or more of the following medications:

Class of medication	Chemical names (some brand names)
Diuretics	Hydrochlorothiazide (Esidrix, Hydrodiuril, Microzide)
	Chlorothiazide (Diuril)
	Chlorthalidone (Hygroton)
	Furosemide (Lasix)
	Spironolactone (Aldactone)
	Triamterene (Dyrenium)
ACE inibitors	Captopril (Capoten)
	Enalapril (Vasotec)
	Ramipril (Altace)
	Lisinopril (Zestril, Prinivil)
	Quinapril (Accupril)
	Fosinopril (Monopril)
	Trandolapril (Mavik)
	Benazepril (Lotensin)
Angiotension II receptor blockers	Losartan (Cozaar)
	Valsartan (Diovan)
	Irbesartan (Avapro)
	Candesartan (Atacand)
Beta blockers	Metoprolol (Lopressor)
	Metoprolol XL (Toprol-XL)
	Atenolol (Tenormin)
	Propranolol (Inderal)
	Sotalol (Betaspace)
	Timilol (Blocadren)
	Acebutolol (Sectral)
	Nadolol (Corgard)
Alpha blockers	Doxazosin mesylate (Cardura)
	Prazosin hydrochloride (Minipress)
	Terazosin hydrochloride (Hytrin)
Combined alpha and beta blockers	Carvediol (Coreg)
	Labetalol (Normodyne, Trandate)
Calcium channel blockers	Amlodipine (Norvasc)
	Diltiazem (Cardizem CD, Cardizem SR, Dilacor XR, Tiazec)
	Nifedipine (Adalat CC, Procardia XL)
	Verapamil hydrochloride (Calan SR, Covera HS, Isoptin SR, Verelan)
Vasodilators	Isosorbide (Imdur, Ismo, Isordil)

blood pressure is not considered high. There is good evidence that ACE inhibitors help delay the further development of kidney disease and cardiovascular disease, unrelated to whether a person has high blood pressure. ARBs are similarly effective in reducing the rate of kidney disease. Your blood pressure should be checked every time you visit the doctor.

IMPROVE YOUR PROFILE: CHOLESTEROL AND TRIGLYCERIDES

The majority of women as well as men with type 2 diabetes also have abnormal cholesterol or triglyceride levels. In 2000, the federal government's Centers for Disease Control and Prevention reported that more than 70 percent of people with diabetes have dyslipidemia, a pattern of abnormal cholesterol and triglyceride readings. Dyslipidemia significantly increases the chance of macrovascular complications and may increase the risk of eye disease.

Cholesterol is a waxy, fatlike substance that the body needs to function properly. It is responsible for forming cell walls and helping to make certain hormones. Low-density lipoproteins (LDLs) carry cholesterol through the bloodstream to where it is needed, and high-density lipoproteins (HDLs) scoop up any excess cholesterol and bring it back to the liver, where cholesterol is made. If LDL cholesterol is high and HDL is low, too much cholesterol remains in the arteries, where it can build up in the artery walls, forming "plaques," which narrow and harden the walls.

When a plaque ruptures in the arterial wall, a blood clot may form at the site, further compromising blood flow. In addition, cholesterol build-up causes inflammation. The end result is arteriosclerosis, which can ultimately block blood flow. Blocked vessels to the heart cause a heart attack. Blocked vessels to the brain cause a stroke. Blocked vessels to the feet and legs cause muscular pain during exercise and can contribute to the development of ulcers that sometimes require amputation.

Triglycerides are also lipids that are transported around the blood system by lipoproteins. The body needs triglycerides for energy, but any excess is stored in fatty tissues. The most familiar storage site is the flabby tissue around the waist and hips. Increased triglyceride levels also contribute to arteriosclerosis in people with diabetes.

HDL cholesterol is a scavenger that helps dispose of excess cholesterol so it will not find its way into vessel walls. In people with diabetes, especially type 2 diabetes, increased triglycerides are often accompanied by low HDL levels, increasing the risk of heart disease.

Thus diabetic dyslipidemia is defined most commonly by

➡ high triglyceride levels;
➡ low HDL levels; and
➡ small, dense LDL particles that even at normal levels can promote build-up of plaque in the arteries.

Losing weight and becoming more physically active are two known ways to reduce triglycerides and increase somewhat the "good" cholesterol and lower the "bad" cholesterol. (See Table 4.2 for more detail on lipid levels.) The tips we included in Chapter 3 for lowering fats in the diet will also help lower cholesterol, as dietary fat and high blood cholesterol often go hand in hand. Remember that the liver produces the cholesterol the body requires, so we don't need to get any cholesterol from the foods we eat. If you need to lower your LDL, you should take in less than 30 percent of your daily calories as fat and reduce saturated fat to less than 10 percent. Reducing cholesterol to less than 200 mg per day will also help. In Chapter 3 we showed you how to read food labels so you can achieve these goals.

Better blood glucose control can also improve HDL and especially triglyceride levels. But medications may be needed for those who cannot reach desired levels of these lipids. LDL levels are generally lower in women than in men until menopause, when levels increase and LDL particles become smaller and denser. In women, changes in HDL and triglyceride levels may be better predictors of cardiovascular

Table 4.2   More of the good, less of the bad

Type of cholesterol (mg/dl)	Classification
LDL	
< 100	Optimal
100–129	Near or above optimal
130–159	Borderline high
160–189	High
≥ 190	Very high
HDL	
< 40	Low
> 40	Desirable in men
≥ 50	Desirable in women
Total cholesterol	
< 200	Desirable
200–239	Borderline high
≥ 240	High
Triglycerides	
< 150	Normal
150–199	Borderline high
200–499	High
> 500	Very high

Source: Adapted from: NCEP-ATP III guidelines (www.nhlbi.nih.gov/guidelines/cholesterol/atp3upd04.htm).

risk than LDL. Treatments that improve all aspects of the lipid profile should be considered. The medicines most often prescribed are the statins, fibrates, and niacin.

Most women with diabetes should set three specific goals:

➡ Lower LDL to less than 100 mg/dl (or to less than 70 mg/dl if you have had a heart attack or are at extremely high risk for heart disease).
➡ Lower triglycerides to less than 150 mg/dl.
➡ Raise HDL to greater than 50 mg/dl (for men, the goal is greater than 40 mg/dl).

Women with type 1 diabetes who maintain good control of their glucose tend to have normal lipid levels, unless they are overweight. In that case, their lipid profiles are often similar to the profiles of women

COMMON CHOLESTEROL-LOWERING MEDICATIONS

HMG CoA reductase inhibitors (statins)
  Atorvastatin (Lipitor)
  Lovastatin (generic)
  Pravastatin (previously Pravachol, now generic)
  Simvastatin (previously Zocor, now generic)
  Fluvastatin (Lescol)
  Rosuvastatin (Crestor)
Bile acid sequestrants
  Cholestyramine (generic packets)
  Questran (cholestyramine) granules
  Colestipol (colestid granules)
  Colestid packets
Niacin
  Niacin (generic)
  Niacin XR (Niaspan)
Fibrates
  Gemfibrozil (generic)
  Fenofibrate (Lofibra, micronized)
  Fenofibrate (Tricor)
Cholesterol absorption inhibitors
  Ezetimibe (Zetia)
Combinations
  Niacin XR and lovastatin (Advicor)
  Simvastatin and Ezetimibe (Vytorin)

with type 2 diabetes. Nonetheless, all women with diabetes should have fasting lipid tests done yearly.

THE NEW YOU

You may have noticed that weight control and physical activity were integral to the three strategies for preventing complications of diabetes. A balanced diet low in saturated fat (but with moderate levels of monosaturated fat, such as that found in olive oil) is desirable. If you spread your carbohydrate intake throughout the day, you can help control blood sugar. Increasing moderate physical activity to thirty minutes or more at least every other day, and daily if possible, helps control weight, blood sugar, and blood pressure.

Everyone with diabetes should receive medical nutrition therapy, a plan preferably developed by a registered dietitian familiar with diabetes (see Chapter 7). The plan will help you reach the desired levels of glucose and HgbA$_{1c}$, cholesterol and triglycerides, blood pressure, and weight. It will guide you in making healthful food choices and integrating exercise into your existing lifestyle.

If you are a cigarette smoker, you know the dangers posed to your health. There is overwhelming evidence linking this habit to heart disease, stroke, and peripheral vascular disease. Quitting decreases this risk substantially (see Chapter 8 for tips on how to do it). Smoking has also been linked to the premature development of microvascular complications of diabetes. Women with diabetes are strongly advised not to smoke.

INCENTIVES FOR CHANGE

Blood glucose control, blood pressure control, and lipid control—these are the three main goals you should strive for. The incentive to reach these goals is the possibility of avoiding the many complications we will now describe.

CARDIOVASCULAR COMPLICATIONS

As many as 75 percent of people with diabetes die from heart disease or stroke. Heart disease is the number one killer of American women, and stroke is number three (after cancer). But if you add diabetes to the equation, the risk of cardiovascular disease goes up as much as fivefold.

Cardiovascular disease includes diseases of the vessel system that circulates blood to the heart, brain, and extremities. It causes heart attacks (also called myocardial infarctions, or MIs, for short) and strokes.

Peripheral vascular disease, which is caused by blockage of the arteries that supply blood to the extremities, most often affects the feet and legs. People with diabetes are seven to nine times more likely than nondiabetics to have peripheral vascular disease. Smoking substantially increases the risk of peripheral vascular disease.

Part of the increased risk for cardiovascular disease in people with type 2 diabetes is explained by high rates of hypertension, dyslipidemia, and obesity, each of which causes arteriosclerosis. In addition, high levels of glucose appear to damage the walls of arteries. And finally, women with diabetes have a particularly high risk for cardiovascular disease compared with nondiabetic women for reasons not well understood. The usual protective effects of estrogen disappear in women with diabetes.

If you already have diabetes, you can't change that fact. But you can adjust your lifestyle to help prevent cardiovascular and peripheral vascular disease by

➡ reducing blood pressure;
➡ reducing lipid levels;

➡ quitting cigarette smoking;

➡ taking a low-dose (81 mg) aspirin daily;

➡ losing weight if you are overweight, and exercising most days of the week; and

➡ reducing blood glucose.

Aspirin therapy is now recommended for people with diabetes as a way to make blood platelet cells less "sticky" and so less likely to clot. Not everyone should take aspirin (those who are allergic to it or have bleeding tendencies should not, for example). By contrast, women with active heart disease may need doses higher than 81 mg. Ask your doctor if you should take aspirin and, if so, how much.

Hormone replacement therapy (HRT) used to be almost routinely recommended for women at menopause to prevent osteoporosis (bone thinning). Estrogens were also thought to reduce heart disease and stroke. However, more recent, definitive studies have shown that hormone replacement therapy may actually increase the risk of heart disease and stroke. Therefore, HRT should only be used for the shortest time necessary to relieve menopausal symptoms. Birth control pills carry little increased risk of cardiovascular disease, unless you have high blood pressure or smoke.

Researchers are also exploring the relationship between depression—which is twice as common in women with diabetes than in women without—and cardiovascular disease. Depression seems to be associated with the development of cardiovascular disease, particularly heart disease, and is related to a poorer outcome after a heart attack. It may be that people with depression are less likely than others to follow recommendations for controlling diabetes and its complications. But depression is also associated with such physiological changes as nervous system activation, heart rhythm disturbances, and inflammation of blood vessels, which may negatively affect the cardiovascular system. We don't yet know if effective treatment of depression reduces the risk of cardiovascular disease.

Heart-Felt Concerns

Deaths from heart disease among women with diabetes have increased 23 percent over the past thirty years or so. Compare this to the fact that such deaths have *decreased* 27 percent in women without diabetes. Although men have more heart attacks and strokes than women, women are more likely to die from them.

Part of the reason for this discrepancy is that women and even their physicians tend to think of heart attacks, or MIs, as something that happens mainly to men. Heart attack symptoms in women can be more subtle than in men, and so women may be less likely to seek immediate help. In addition, physicians don't treat the risk factors as aggressively in women as in men. What we do know is that women, particularly those with diabetes, should be vigilant about what's happening to their bodies.

Coronary artery disease affects the blood vessels supplying the heart and is the most common form of heart disease. It includes angina (chest pain) and heart attacks, and results in heart failure, disability, and death. Age is a major risk factor, and women over the age of forty, with or without diabetes, are at greater risk for heart disease than younger women. But once diagnosed with diabetes, a woman is at such increased risk that, to reduce risk factors, she should be treated medically as if she already has coronary heart disease.

If you have diabetes, your physician should assess your risk factors for coronary heart disease every year and prescribe medication if necessary. High blood pressure and dyslipidemia should be treated aggressively. If you smoke, stop. Depending on your risk profile, you may need a cardiac stress test or some other diagnostic screening test. Women tend to have more false-positive results on exercise stress tests than men (meaning that the test is positive, but subsequent, more definitive tests do not reveal clinically significant heart disease). For this reason your physician may order an imaging test, or echocardiogram, to assess the distribution of blood flow and cardiac function in response to exercise.

Women should be aware of the signs of a heart attack, which can be different from what men experience. Diabetes can also change the presentation of the symptoms of heart disease. Heart attacks are often not as dramatic as they appear in the movies, with someone clutching his chest and collapsing. Many heart attacks start out slowly with mild pain, a pressing, squeezing sense of discomfort, jaw pain, or only shortness of breath.

Here are the signs you should be aware of, according to the American Heart Association:

➡ chest discomfort or uncomfortable pressure, squeezing, fullness, or pain. The feeling can last longer than a few minutes or can come and go. This is the most common symptom for women and men;

➡ discomfort in other areas of the upper body: in one or both arms, the back, neck, jaw, or stomach;

➡ shortness of breath: this can occur before or along with chest discomfort; and

➡ lightheadedness, nausea, or breaking into a cold sweat.

Women are somewhat more likely than men to have shortness of breath, nausea, vomiting, and back or jaw pain. Women are also more likely to have a "silent MI," that is, a heart attack they never knew they had. If you or someone you are with has one or more of the above symptoms, no matter how subtle, stop what you are doing and call 911 immediately.

Blood Flow to the Brain

Having diabetes also puts you at a much greater risk of having a stroke, the brain's version of a heart attack. People with diabetes are also more likely than nondiabetics to be left with a permanent disability or to have a poor chance for survival after a stroke.

A stroke occurs most commonly when there is a sudden lack of blood flow to some part of the brain, usually because a blood vessel has been clogged through atherosclerosis (fatty deposits that harden the arteries) or because a clot or bleeding occurs in the abnormal vessels.

Brain tissue needs a constant supply of oxygen and nutrients provided by the bloodstream. If the supply is cut off for longer than four minutes, tissue in the part of the brain supplied by the blocked-off vessels begins to die.

Since the various areas of the brain have specialized functions, the losses experienced by someone after a stroke depend on what area of the brain was damaged and the extent of the damage. Stroke may cause one side of the body to be paralyzed or weakened, or can result in memory problems, trouble speaking or understanding speech, problems with eating or swallowing, and difficulty balancing.

Someone who is having a stroke or a "transient ischemic attack" (a warning sign of a stroke with symptoms that last only a few minutes to hours) must get to the hospital immediately. Tests will determine if what the person is experiencing is indeed a stroke. If it is, she will most likely be given blood clot–busting drugs. These drugs must be given within three hours of the start of a stroke to be most effective, which is why time is of the essence.

Signs of a stroke are usually sudden and include:

➡ numbness or weakness of the face, arm, or leg, especially on one side of the body;
➡ confusion, trouble speaking or understanding;
➡ trouble seeing in one or both eyes, or double vision;
➡ trouble walking, lack of balance, or dizziness; and
➡ severe headache with no known cause.

And Flow to the Toe

A common and severe, but often unnoticed, vascular complication of diabetes is peripheral vascular disease (PVD; also called peripheral arterial disease). It is caused by arteriosclerosis, in this case, the narrowing and stiffening of the arteries that supply the leg with blood. It is estimated that one-third of people with diabetes over age fifty have PVD, but many don't know it. Often there are no symptoms or only subtle ones, such as leg pain or fatigue while walking, which people may in-

Table 4.3   Warning signs of foot problems

Cause	Symptoms	Findings during physical exam
Circulation	Cold feet; pain with walking, usually in calf or foot, but may also affect thighs and buttocks	Little or no pulses felt by doctor in lower extremities; red feet when sitting or standing; low skin temperature
Nerve damage	Burning, tingling, or sensation like ants crawling on skin; pain and discomfort with light touch; decrease in sweating	Loss of sensation to light touch or vibration most common; decreased ankle reflexes; more rarely, loss of strength
Muscle problems	Change in foot shape; swelling	Claw-like toes
Skin problems	Slow-healing wounds; blue or deep-red skin; scaly, itchy feet; infections such as ingrown toenails and athlete's foot	Dry, scaly skin; loss of hair on involved area; thickened nails

Source: Adapted from M. Moser and S. Sowers, *Clinical Management of Cardiovascular Risk Factors in Diabetes* (New York: Professional Communications, Inc., 2002).

correctly dismiss as signs that they are getting older. (See Table 4.3 for some warning signs of PVD.)

Screening for PVD is strongly recommended for anyone with diabetes who is over age fifty. PVD is associated with greater risk of heart attacks and stroke, and can result in foot ulcers and lower-extremity amputations. Risk factors for PVD are largely the same as for heart disease and stroke, with smoking playing a particularly dangerous role. Peripheral vascular disorder is often detected by a physical examination. PVD is suspected when peripheral pulses are weak or absent and decreased blood flow results in cool toes or feet, thinning of skin, or loss of hair over the toes and feet. A simple test called the ankle brachial index, which measures blood pressure in a person's ankle compared with blood pressure in the arm, can also identify the disorder. If ankle blood pressure is lower than pressure in the arm, you may have PVD.

Although most often there are no signs of peripheral vascular disease, you should report the following symptoms or problems to your doctor:

➡ leg pain—usually in the calf, thigh, or buttocks—that comes on after you've walked for a relatively short distance (for example, one-half to two blocks), and that resolves after you rest for a few minutes;

➡ slow-healing sores or infections on the feet or legs.

Checking your feet

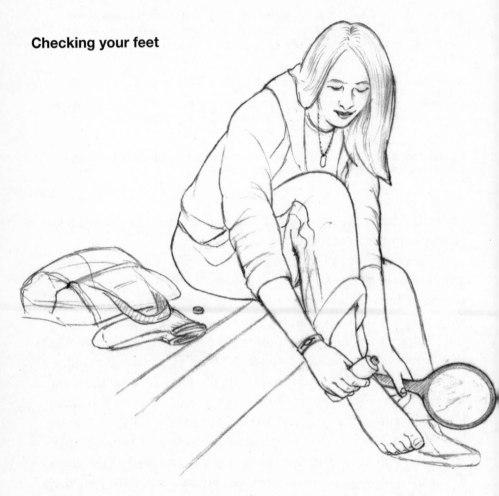

Inspect your feet and toes daily for cuts, blisters, redness, calluses, or swelling. A mirror will help you see the bottom of your feet. Moisturize, but don't get the lotion in between your toes. (See pages 104–105 for more tips.)

The following interventions are particularly useful in slowing or reversing the disease process:

➡ Stop smoking immediately.
➡ Walk as much as your symptoms allow.
➡ Take aspirin or other medications to decrease clotting of blood.
➡ In more advanced cases, talk to your doctor about procedures to unblock or bypass blocked vessels.

The Microvascular Complications

We've shown you what can happen if medium- or large-sized arteries—the "macro" vessels—get blocked and how to stop this from happening. The other complications that are more specific to diabetes result from damage to the "micro," or small, blood vessels—the capillaries—that feed various parts of the body, including the eyes and the kidneys. High blood pressure and abnormal lipid levels do contribute to these disease processes too, but microvascular complications are primarily caused by long-term exposure to high blood sugar.

The studies described earlier in this chapter showed the clear benefits of maintaining blood glucose levels as close to normal levels as safely possible. Careful blood pressure control also reduces the risk of microvascular complications. Screening for the early changes of microvascular and neurologic complications can identify problems before they become major clinical events—such as loss of vision, kidney failure, and amputations—and while there is still time to prevent them.

The following strategies help detect early microvascular complications:

➡ yearly eye exams
➡ yearly kidney function tests
➡ regular foot exams at all doctor visits (in addition to routine foot care at home)
➡ regular dental checks for gum disease (at least annually)

If screening tests detect early complications, effective interventions can delay their progression.

KEEP AN EYE ON PROBLEMS

Yearly eye exams are a good idea for everyone over age forty but are critical if you have diabetes. Certain eye diseases like cataracts (clouding of the lens of the eye) and glaucoma (build-up of fluid pressure within the eye) are much more common as we get older and are even more common in those who have diabetes. But the most pressing reason for yearly exams is to catch the early stages of diabetic retinopathy—when sight can still be saved. The longer you've had diabetes, the greater your risk of retinopathy.

Diabetic retinopathy occurs when the tiny blood vessels inside the retina—the tissue at the back of the eye that senses light and sends images to the brain—become damaged. In the early stages of the disease, the vessels leak fluid and balloon out, causing small lesions called microaneurysms. There are usually no symptoms at this early stage. The only way to detect this early stage, called background retinopathy or nonproliferative diabetic retinopathy, is with an eye examination or by photographing the back of the eye.

But if the leakage occurs in or near the small area of the retina called the macula, the area responsible for fine-detailed central vision, sight may be affected. This so-called diabetic macular edema can happen at any time after the diagnosis of diabetes, but rarely occurs until someone has had diabetes for at least five years.

Retinopathy may or may not progress to the next, more serious stage called proliferative diabetic retinopathy. As time goes on, the small vessels become blocked, depriving the eye of its blood supply. New blood vessels are stimulated to grow. These new vessels are abnormal and very fragile, however, so they bleed easily. They may bleed into the vitreous, the normally clear gel-like material that fills the inner eye. This in turn may cause a build-up of scar tissue that pulls on the retina and detaches it. Or the abnormal blood vessels may stop the flow of fluid out of the eye and cause pressure to build up, resulting in a form of glaucoma called neovascular glaucoma.

Most vision loss can be prevented if retinopathy is detected early

The retina in diabetes

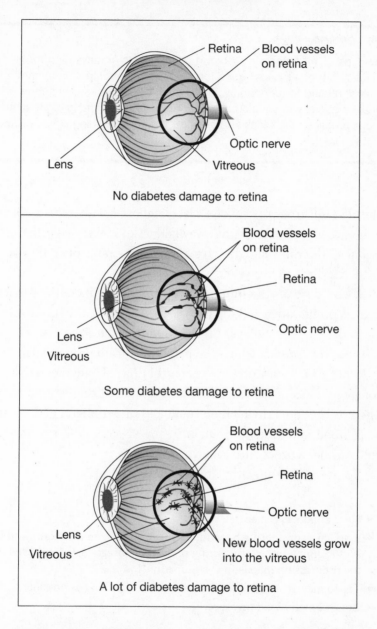

Retina
Blood vessels on retina
Optic nerve
Vitreous
Lens

No diabetes damage to retina

Blood vessels on retina
Retina
Optic nerve
Lens
Vitreous

Some diabetes damage to retina

Blood vessels on retina
Retina
Optic nerve
New blood vessels grow into the vitreous
Lens
Vitreous

A lot of diabetes damage to retina

The retina is the tissue at the back of the eye that sends images to the brain. In diabetic retinopathy, the tiny blood vessels inside the retina become damaged. Most of the time, loss of sight can be prevented if problems are detected early. (National Institute of Diabetes and Digestive and Kidney Diseases; http://diabetes.niddk.nih.gov/dm/pubs/complications_eyes/index.htm#5.)

SIGHT FOR SORE EYES

Sometimes vision gets blurry if blood sugar spikes or stays high for a while (it can also happen if sugar goes too low). This is a temporary change only and is not related to retinopathy. However, if the blurriness lasts more than a couple of days, you should call your doctor. Other warning signs of severe eye problems are black spots called "floaters," flashing lights, or any loss of vision.

in the disease process. Anyone just diagnosed with type 2 diabetes should have an eye exam right away and at least every year thereafter. Someone with type 1 should have annual eye exams once they've had diabetes for three to five years.

If you develop the more severe forms of retinopathy—macular edema or proliferative retinopathy—laser therapy, which burns small areas in the back of the eye, can be used to reduce the rate of vision loss. These treatments, which are performed in the eye specialist's office, do not usually restore any vision that has already been lost. The major side effects of the extensive laser treatment that is used to treat proliferative retinopathy include some loss of peripheral and night vision. If blood and scarring remain in the vitreous, the eye specialist might consider a procedure called a vitrectomy.

To prevent retinopathy and its consequences:

➡ Have annual eye exams.
➡ If you are considering becoming pregnant, have an eye exam; and have eyes examined regularly during pregnancy (pregnancy may speed up the progression of existing retinopathy).
➡ Try to maintain tight blood glucose control as long as possible.
➡ Control high blood pressure.

KIDNEY CONCERNS

Kidney disease (nephropathy) is another serious complication of diabetes; it affects 20 to 40 percent of people with type 1 and type 2 diabetes. Blood vessel changes within the kidney can compromise its ability to filter wastes. The first sign that the kidney's filtration system is being damaged is microalbuminuria, the presence of tiny amounts of a protein called albumin in the urine. Often people with type 2 diabetes who have microalbuminuria also have hypertension. Microalbuminuria is also a predictor of cardiovascular disease.

Without treatment, most people with type 1 diabetes who have microalbuminuria will advance through the stages of nephropathy, and about 75 percent of them will develop end-stage renal disease, or total kidney failure, after about twenty years. Once the kidneys have failed, dialysis (a procedure for removing wastes from the blood) or a kidney transplant are the only options. Those with type 2 diabetes are less likely than those with type 1 to end up with kidney failure after twenty years, but that's probably because in the past most of them died from cardiovascular disease first.

In the early stages, diabetic kidney disease usually has no symptoms and can be detected only with blood creatinine and urine albumin testing. But as toxic wastes build up in the body, people with severe kidney disease may feel nauseated and vomit, lose their appetites, and gain weight as a result of fluid retention. Untreated, fluid can fill the lungs and result in heart failure.

Tight blood glucose control and blood pressure control have been shown to prevent or at least slow the development of microalbuminuria and its progression to advanced kidney disease. If your physician discovers microalbuminuria, he or she may start you on an angiotensin-coverting enzyme (ACE) inhibitor or angiotensin II receptor blocker (ARB), if you are not already taking one, to protect the kidneys. Weight loss, exercise, and reduced salt and alcohol consumption are also recommended. In addition, a dietitian may suggest that you reduce the amount of protein in your diet.

LOSING YOUR NERVE

Small blood vessels also supply nerves with oxygen and nutrients. Decreased blood flow to the nerves and other chemical changes associated with high blood glucose levels contribute to nerve damage (neuropathy).

The nervous system is a massive information highway that branches out from the brain and spinal cord to all parts of the body. The damage resulting from diabetes usually occurs in the peripheral nervous system, which carries sensory information (hot/cold, pain, and other sensations) from various parts of the body to the brain, and carries nerve impulses that control the muscles of the extremities. Diabetes can also affect the autonomic nervous system, which supplies the automatic muscles of the heart, bladder, stomach, intestines, and sexual organs.

The symptoms of peripheral and autonomic neuropathy depend on which nerves are affected. The most common complaint resulting from neuropathy is a pins and needles sensation, numbness, or tingling in the legs or feet. Women with diabetes may suffer from carpal tunnel syndrome, in which the nerve running from the forearm into the hand becomes compressed and causes numbness, weakness, or pain in parts of the hand. Someone with neuropathy may have no symptoms, or symptoms so mild that they go unnoticed for many years. Other, less common symptoms include

➡ loss of balance;
➡ pain in the legs, usually at night and at rest (different from the muscular pain with walking that occurs with peripheral vascular disease);
➡ indigestion, nausea, vomiting, diarrhea, or constipation;
➡ inability to empty the bladder;
➡ frequent urinary tract infections;
➡ painless foot ulcers (open sores) or lack of pain sensation from foot injuries.

Here again, the best prevention is to maintain tight glucose control, which can reduce your risk of neuropathy by at least half. People with neuropathy also have to pay particular attention to their feet. The nerves to the feet are the longest in the body and the ones most often

SYMPTOMS OF NERVE DAMAGE CAUSED BY DIABETES

Peripheral nerve problems (nerves not located in the brain or spinal cord)

Toes, feet, legs, hands, and arms	Numbness (pins and needles)
	Tingling or burning sensations
	Extreme sensitivity to touch or insensitivity to light touch, vibration, or temperature
	Loss of balance and coordination
	Muscle weakness

Autonomic nerve problems (the nerves that regulate heart rate, blood pressure, perspiration, bladder function, and digestion)

Heart, gut, urinary system, sweat glands, and eyes	Low blood pressure and dizziness when standing up
	Irregular heart rate
	Wide fluctuations in blood sugar
	Chronic constipation or diarrhea
	Difficulty emptying stomach—unusual fullness after meals
	Decreased sexual response
	Chronic urinary tract infections
	Incontinence (spontaneous loss of urine)
	Abnormal sweating

affected by neuropathy. Nerve damage can lead to ulcers that become infected and require amputation of a toe, foot, or lower limb. (See Table 4.4 for treatment of nerve conditions resulting from diabetes.)

One in four people with diabetes develops foot problems—at the extreme, the damage is so severe that amputation is required. You are at increased risk for diabetic foot problems if you have neuropathy and

Tight glucose control can reduce your risk of nerve damage by at least half.

Table 4.4 Treating conditions related to neuropathy

Condition	Treatment
Foot ulcers	Take care of wound; keep weight off foot, sometimes using contact casting; surgical removal of the damaged tissue; antibiotics; hyperbaric treatment to heal the tissue
Pain	Over-the-counter pain medications; specific neuropathy medications; avoid narcotics if possible; nerve stimulation; electrotherapy; acupuncture
Nerve entrapment such as carpal tunnel syndrome	Splinting and rest of the limb involved; local corticosteroid injection; over-the-counter anti-inflammatory medications, such as Advil or Naprosyn; surgical repair

Source: Adapted from National Institute of Diabetes, Digestive, and Kidney Disease website, 2003 (http://win.niddk.nih.gov).

peripheral vascular disease. Everyone with diabetes should receive regular foot examinations, ideally at every medical office visit.

If you have lost feeling in your feet as a result of advanced neuropathy, you might not notice if calluses or blisters from poorly fitted shoes become infected. If these infections are not discovered early enough or if treatment is unsuccessful, ulcers can develop.

Once someone has a foot ulcer, every effort must be made to try to heal it. Usually this means staying off your feet to relieve the pressure and seeing a specialist such as a podiatrist or vascular surgeon to remove any infected tissue. Total contact casts, which fit around the entire foot, may be used to relieve pressure over ulcers. In difficult cases when the ulcers are not healing, physicians might use "living skin equivalents" to cover the wound, or topical growth factors to encourage healing of the tissue. Vascular surgery may be done to improve circulation to the foot if the patient has peripheral vascular disease. As the options for treatment have increased, amputation has become much rarer. In fact, with proper care of the feet, the risk of amputation can be cut in half.

Here are some steps to follow at home to prevent foot problems:

➡ Wash your feet daily with warm, not hot, water; dry them thoroughly, particularly between the toes.

➡ Inspect your feet and toes daily for cuts, blisters, redness, calluses, or swelling. Use a mirror to see the bottom of your feet, and get prompt treatment if you notice anything new. (See page 96.)

➡ Moisturize your feet with lotion, but don't get the lotion between your toes.

➡ Never walk barefooted.

➡ Cut your toenails to the gently rounded shape of your toes and file the edges with an emery board; don't remove calluses yourself.

➡ Wear shoes that fit well, cushioned by thick, soft socks or pressure-relieving insoles. New shoes should fit well and not cause damage from friction. You shouldn't need to break in new shoes.

➡ Before putting on your shoes, inspect them to make sure there is nothing inside them and no sharp edges that could injure your feet.

KEEP TEETH INTACT

If you have been diagnosed with diabetes, you should let your dentist know. Periodontal disease (bacterial infection in the gums, which anchor our teeth) is more likely to occur in someone with diabetes who has not controlled blood glucose levels very well. Increased glucose levels in saliva feed the bacteria in our mouths, which sets the stage for gum disease. Risk is also increased as blood vessels narrow, slowing the flow of nutrients into the mouth and the outflow of wastes from the mouth.

Periodontal disease starts with plaque build-up on the teeth, which irritates the gums and causes bleeding. Left unchecked, periodontitis destroys bone and connective tissue, causing teeth to become loose. If you have diabetes, there are two very good reasons to take care of your gums: not only is diabetes a risk factor for periodontal disease, but periodontal disease may make diabetes worse.

Treating periodontal disease is particularly important if you are pregnant or planning to become pregnant. Some women experience bleeding or swollen gums during pregnancy, but if you have diabetes, gum problems can be much more serious.

To prevent periodontal disease, the American Academy of Periodontology recommends:

➡ tight glucose control;

➡ brushing and flossing daily to remove plaque (your dentist can recommend special mouthwashes, electric toothbrushes, and toothpastes to reduce plaque and control infection);

➡ professional cleaning at least twice a year (more frequently if disease is already present), along with an evaluation for the presence of disease.

SKIN CHANGES

When blood glucose runs high, your body loses fluid and your skin can become dry. Another cause of dry, itchy skin is neuropathy. The nerves in the legs and feet may not get the message to sweat, a process that keeps skin moist.

Other skin problems can occur along with diabetes because high blood glucose can be a breeding ground for bacteria and fungi. Most of these skin problems can be prevented or readily treated if caught early, before they become more serious. See Table 4.5 for skin conditions common in people with diabetes.

ACUTE METABOLIC COMPLICATIONS OF DIABETES

Three emergency, potentially life-threatening situations can result if glucose levels are very high or too low. Friends and family members should become acquainted with the warning signs of these conditions so they can come to your assistance if necessary.

Diabetic ketoacidosis (DKA) occurs when stores of insulin are severely depleted and levels of glucose rise unchecked. DKA usually happens only when someone has not been following her insulin therapy, and it is often triggered by an illness or infection, such as pneumonia or a urinary tract infection. DKA can also be triggered by a heart attack or stroke, or some other severe illness or injury to the body. DKA is much more common in those with type 1 diabetes than in those with type 2 diabetes, where it occurs rarely.

DKA results when, in the absence of adequate insulin, blood glu-

Table 4.5   Common skin problems related to diabetes

Diabetic dermopathy
- Occurs in 10–30 percent of those with diabetes
- Pigmented spots most commonly seen over the tibia (shin) bone of the lower leg
- Clinical significance not clear

Necrobiosis lipoidica diabeticorum (NLD)
- Rare, but more frequent in women between ages 30 and 40
- Red bumps that develop into irregular red thickened patches with a yellow center; can ulcerate and become painful
- Occur most commonly on legs
- May resolve spontaneously

Bullosis diabeticorum
- Rare
- Large blisters on top of feet and toes
- More common in men
- Often resolves spontaneously

Granuloma annulare
- Can be local or generalized
- Usually seen between ages 30 and 70
- Round, flesh-colored rash usually on upper trunk, neck, and arms
- Topical corticosteroid cream can help

Acanthosis nigricans
- Rough, velvety dark patches on back of neck
- Indicative of a high degree of insulin resistance
- May be reduced by weight loss

---

cose rises to very high levels, leading to dehydration. In addition, fat stores start dissolving and the body produces waste products called ketones. The dehydration and accumulation of ketones create a highly acidic state. DKA is uncommon in type 2 diabetes because in that form of the disease the body is still able to produce some insulin, which prevents ketones from accumulating.

Ketones can be detected in urine with a simple dipstick test performed at home. Women with diabetes, particularly type 1 diabetes, should check for urine ketones if blood sugar levels are high (greater than 300) for more than eight hours, or if they have nausea, vomiting,

SYMPTOMS OF DIABETIC KETOACIDOSIS

If you have type 1 diabetes, you are at risk for diabetic ketoacidosis (DKA). DKA rarely occurs in type 2 diabetes. DKA can happen if you skip insulin injections or if your body requires more insulin than you are taking, for example, when you're sick. Be aware of the symptoms of DKA and call your health care provider immediately if you have any of them:

Symptoms of severe hyperglycemia (high blood sugar):

- Increased urination
- Thirst
- Dry mouth

Very high blood glucose levels (greater than 300 mg/dl)

Fruity-smelling breath

Nausea or vomiting

Abdominal pain

Confusion

Ketones in the urine or blood

---

abdominal pain, or a fever over 100 degrees. DKA requires emergency treatment in a hospital to correct the imbalances of fluid, insulin, and electrolytes, such as sodium and potassium.

Hyperosmolar hyperglycemic, nonketotic coma is another acute complication of high glucose levels. It is much more common in type 2 than in type 1 diabetes. Some of the symptoms of hyperosmolar coma are similar to those of DKA, however. The main difference is that glucose levels are usually higher in hyperosmolar coma and result in increasing confusion, sleepiness, and, if not treated, coma. In addition, ketoacidosis is not present. The condition requires immediate medical attention for intravenous fluids and insulin to control the high blood sugar. Hyperosmolar hyperglycemic coma occurs mainly in older people with type 2 diabetes. It is sometimes the first indication that someone has diabetes.

Hypoglycemia results when blood glucose falls below a critical

SYMPTOMS OF HYPEROSMOLAR HYPERGLYCEMIA

If you have type 2 diabetes, extremely high levels of blood glucose (usually more than 600 mg/dl) can result in a life-threatening condition called hyperosmolar hyperglycemia. It can happen when you are ill, have an infection, are dehydrated, or miss your medication. You need to call your health care provider immediately if you have any of the following symptoms:

Symptoms of severe hyperglycemia (high blood sugar):

- Increased urination
- Thirst
- Dry mouth

Very high blood glucose (greater than 600 mg/dl)

Dehydration and dizziness

Confusion

level, usually less than 70 mg/dl. It occurs in people treated with insulin or sulfonylureas (a commonly prescribed oral diabetes medication that increases insulin secretion) when they have too much insulin, not enough food, unanticipated exercise, or a combination of these factors. Hypoglycemia is usually mild and can be remedied by eating or drinking something containing carbohydrates to raise blood sugars. But if left untreated, hypoglycemia can lead to unconsciousness or seizures, so early recognition and treatment are important.

Early warning signs of hypoglycemia include nervousness, perspiration, shakiness, and a fast heartbeat. If not treated, glucose levels drop further and can result in confusion, sleepiness, difficulty thinking, seizures, and loss of consciousness.

People with type 1 diabetes who use intensive insulin therapy have an increased risk of hypoglycemia. (Hypoglycemia can also happen, although less frequently, to people with type 2 diabetes who are treated with insulin or sulfonylurea drugs to lower glucose.) Sometimes, despite your best efforts, glucose levels dip too low. This can happen if you skip a meal or have a smaller meal than planned. Hypo-

WHAT TO DO WHEN YOUR BLOOD SUGAR DROPS

You should always have some quick-fix foods on hand in a purse or at your bedside for those times when your glucose drops too low: 5 or 6 pieces of hard candy, 2 or 3 glucose tablets, 1/2 cup (4 ounces) of fruit juice, 1/2 cup of regular (not diet) soft drink, or 1 or 2 teaspoons of sugar or honey. Fifteen minutes after taking one serving, measure your blood sugar again. If it's still not up to at least 70 mg/dl, have another serving. Repeat these steps until your blood glucose level is up to at least 70 mg/dl. If your next meal won't be for an hour or more, you might also have a more substantial snack. You will need emergency care only if you are too confused to eat or drink a sugar-containing food, or if you lose consciousness.

glycemia can also be related to more intensive exercise on a given day, too large a dose of insulin, your menstrual cycle, an illness, excessive alcohol, or other factors your health care team can help you identify and understand. Recognizing the circumstances that lead to hypoglycemia can help you prevent the next episode. Rapid, effective treatment of hypoglycemia will prevent episodes from becoming severe.

To avoid low blood sugar:

➡ Check your glucose levels as recommended by your health care provider.

➡ Check blood sugar before and after you exercise. Eat a snack if your blood sugar is less than 100 mg/dl.

➡ Check your blood sugar before driving a car or operating heavy equipment.

➡ Take your medications as directed.

➡ Don't skip meals.

➡ Try to eat on a regular schedule; if you can't, test your glucose level more frequently.

➡ Carry juice, hard candies, and other "quick-fix" foods at all times.

➡ If you drink alcohol, make sure it is with a meal.

➡ Have glucagon (an injection that raises blood sugar quickly) available at home and at work, and make sure someone close to you knows how to use it.

TAKE-HOME MESSAGE

With diabetes, you will have to pay strict attention to your diet, exercise, blood sugar monitoring, and medications. You will have to visit doctors more frequently and take more medicines than the average person. But you hold the key to controlling the disease and remaining healthy.

You've just read about all the frightening things that can happen if your blood sugars, blood pressure, and lipids are high for long periods of time. But you've also learned what you can do to prevent or delay these medical complications. They are not inevitable. But you must take advantage of what research has shown us. If you follow the strategies outlined in this chapter, you have an excellent shot at reducing your risk of complications from diabetes.

5

Reproductive Health and Sexuality

Maria is twenty-four weeks pregnant and very excited that her obstetrician feels her pregnancy is progressing well. It has been a challenge to perform glucose fingersticks five times a day and take insulin injections for her diabetes, but she is committed to having a healthy pregnancy. She has learned that the more closely she monitors her diabetes and controls her blood sugars, the better her chances of having a healthy baby.

In the past, a discussion of health issues for women with diabetes focused almost exclusively on pregnancy and childbirth. While a healthy pregnancy and child are certainly central concerns, they are by no means the only issues facing women with diabetes. For some women, control of glucose levels can be particularly challenging at certain times in their menstrual cycle, for example. When blood glucose levels run high, yeast, vaginal, and bladder infections are more common. An abnormal balance of calcium, which is more common in diabetes, may increase the risk of bone loss or osteoporosis. Diabetes raises a host of issues for women at menopause and can impact sexuality in a number of ways. Thus at different stages of life, women with diabetes face unique challenges.

DIABETES IN ADOLESCENCE

Although rates of type 2 diabetes are increasing in younger women, type 1 diabetes is still the most common form of the disease among adolescents. Teenage girls with diabetes should be aware that their menstrual periods might start a year or so later than the average for girls without diabetes. In type 1 diabetes, menarche may be delayed because blood glucose levels have not been well controlled, resulting in weight loss. In other cases a problem with thyroid function may be to blame. Though still rare in adolescents, type 2 diabetes may coexist with obesity or a condition called polycystic ovary syndrome (PCOS), both of which can alter normal periods.

Blood glucose levels are particularly difficult to control in the adolescent years of surging hormones. For one thing, the increased production of growth hormone during puberty, which stimulates the development of bone and muscles, interferes with insulin action and increases the need for insulin.

In the best of circumstances, teenagers struggle to assert their independence, come to terms with their sexual identity and body image, and deal with peer pressure and the increased importance of friendships and acceptance. Throw a diagnosis of type 1 or type 2 diabetes into the mix, and the challenges of adolescence increase significantly. Rebellion is common and can center on diabetes care. Teens often take over the management of their diabetes from parents, and strict control does not always result.

For example, girls with type 1 diabetes quickly discover that by skipping insulin doses or taking smaller doses than prescribed they can lose weight quickly. For many teens, the desire to be as thin as a model can be so strong that they are willing to cope with the unpleasant symptoms and long-term consequences of poor diabetes control. Teenagers with diabetes are even more susceptible than other teenage girls to depression, body-image problems, and eating disorders (see next chapter).

Teenagers generally live in the moment. Many of them are more worried about what other teens think of them than about the effect their actions today have on their future health. They want to be like everyone else, and sometimes the "public face" of diabetes self-care—the testing, injections, schedules, and dietary restrictions—may intensify their feelings of being different. They don't always want to think about measuring their blood glucose levels, taking insulin, and making smart food choices. They want to stop for pizza and cokes, stay up late, and maybe drink alcohol. They don't want to worry that a boy or girl will not like them because they have a disease. As a result, teens don't always make the right choices. Occasional lapses in diabetes care are understandable, but parents or health care professionals may have to intervene if noncompliance becomes a self-destructive pattern.

We know that the beneficial effects of intensive therapy are greatest when it is begun early in the disease. The DCCT study, discussed in Chapter 4, clearly established that early, intensive therapy more significantly reduces the risk of eye, nerve, and kidney complications than delayed intervention.

THE MENSTRUAL CYCLE AND GLUCOSE CONTROL

From the start of menstruation until its end at menopause, women have other hormones besides just insulin to consider when keeping blood glucose in the target range. Two of the hormones that control

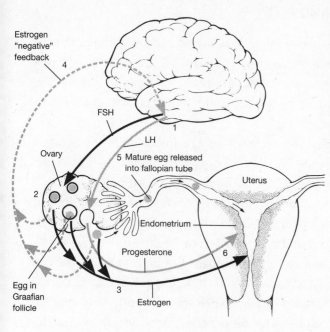

The normal menstrual cycle

The monthly menstrual cycle is driven by hormones. The brain's pituitary gland releases FSH, a hormone that stimulates the ovary to grow a follicle that will "nest" an egg, and releases LH, a hormone that stimulates the ovary to release estrogen. This starts the feedback process that results in estrogen and progesterone's preparing the uterus to receive a fertilized egg. If fertilization does not occur, estrogen and progesterone levels fall, and the thickened, blood-rich lining of the uterus is shed—menstruation.

Estrogen "negative" feedback

4

FSH

1

LH

Ovary

5 Mature egg released into fallopian tube

Uterus

2

Endometrium

Progesterone

6

Egg in Graafian follicle

3

Estrogen

Some women have trouble controlling their diabetes around the time of their period. (K. J. Carlson, S. A. Eisenstat, and T. Ziporyn, *The New Harvard Guide to Women's Health* [Cambridge, Mass.: Harvard University Press, 2004], p. 380.)

the menstrual cycle—estrogen and progesterone—can also affect blood glucose levels. Many women with either type 1 or type 2 diabetes report a significant rise in blood glucose just before their menstrual periods and then a dramatic drop once menstruation begins. Other women don't notice any difference at all.

Menstrual hormones—along with eating habits, exercise, weight change, alcohol, and the dosage of insulin and other medications—are part of a woman's high-wire act of maintaining blood glucose levels as near to normal as possible. Although we don't know exactly why some women have trouble controlling their diabetes around the time of their periods, we do know quite a bit about the menstrual cycle and the interplay of hormones.

HORMONES EBB AND FLOW

The average woman's menstrual cycle is twenty-eight days long, though it can range from twenty-three days to thirty-five. The purpose of this monthly cycle is to prepare a woman's body for possible pregnancy. The cycle is largely driven by the ebb and flow of the hormones estrogen and progesterone.

In the first half of the cycle, called the follicular phase because the egg follicle is maturing, the level of estrogen rises and helps the lining of the uterus grow and thicken. About midway through the cycle, a mature egg leaves one of the ovaries in a process called ovulation. In the second half of the cycle, the luteal phase, the egg travels through the fallopian tube to the uterus. Progesterone begins to rise and works in concert with estrogen to further prepare the uterine lining for potential implantation of a fertilized egg. If the egg is not fertilized, meaning that pregnancy does not occur, the ovaries abruptly stop making estrogen and progesterone. The drop in hormone levels causes the thickened lining of the uterus to shed. This is menstruation.

It is during the luteal phase, when levels of both estrogen and progesterone are highest, that most women report changes in their usual glucose levels. In one survey of 406 women with type 1 diabetes, 67 percent reported changes in blood glucose control before their periods. Women who said they had premenstrual syndrome (PMS) and those who said they had a craving for sweets were particularly likely to experience these changes.

High levels of female hormones appear to be one reason for the change in blood glucose. Some researchers theorize that high levels of progesterone cause a temporary resistance to insulin, which in turn leads to higher glucose levels unless insulin doses are raised. Women with type 2 diabetes tend to be overweight, another factor associated with insulin resistance. High estrogen levels, by contrast, can increase a cell's sensitivity to insulin. The more effectively the body utilizes insulin, the lower the glucose levels will be.

We are not sure why changing levels of hormones affect one

woman differently from another. However, the blood glucose patterns that any one woman experiences often repeat themselves with each cycle, so the more you understand your own pattern, the better you can deal with it.

Even women without diabetes experience changes in their body's reaction to insulin before and during menstruation. But in nondiabetic women, insulin secretion automatically responds to any imbalance, keeping blood sugar levels stable. The body chemistry in someone with diabetes is more precariously balanced, and even slight effects of estrogen and progesterone may throw it off.

Another reason for loss of glucose control may be women's tendency to eat more sweets or carbohydrates before their periods. Women also tend to exercise less if they feel bloated and irritable in the days before their periods begin.

CHART A NEW COURSE

Whatever the reason for glucose fluctuations during the menstrual cycle, your best defense is to know yourself. If you are still menstruating, record your blood glucose levels and medication doses over the next three months, marking down when your period begins. See if there is a pattern: are your blood glucose levels high or low the week before your period or during your period? If you take insulin, have you been requiring more before your period? You might also note any food cravings you indulged in and the time you exercised. Of course, determining a pattern will be easier if your periods are regular. While many women are like clockwork, others have irregular periods, and for them figuring out any patterns will be a challenge.

Once you discover your particular pattern, you and your medical team can tweak your diet plan, exercise regimen, or insulin dosages to keep your glucose levels in a healthy range. Some women need to alter their dose of insulin before dinner or bedtime for two to three days before their periods to reduce high readings first thing in the morning. Often it is this fasting blood glucose that varies the most from one phase of the menstrual cycle to another. Increasing exercise on high-glucose days may be enough to correct your pattern.

If your blood glucose tends to be low on certain days, it might help to adjust your insulin doses or increase carbohydrates preemptively. Knowing what effect, if any, your menstrual cycle has on blood glucose is another piece to the puzzle of maintaining control.

PMS: PREMENSTRUAL SYNDROME

Women who have PMS appear to be especially susceptible to monthly difficulties in blood glucose control. Sometimes relieving the symptoms of PMS is enough to get glucose levels back in line. Symptoms of premenstrual syndrome are both emotional and physical. They generally start a week or so before menstruation and subside when it starts. Some common symptoms are breast tenderness, headaches, water retention (feeling bloated), moodiness, irritability, anxiety or depression, fatigue, difficulty concentrating or remembering, food cravings, and feeling like murdering one's unsympathetic partner. For most women, however, these symptoms are fairly mild and are eased by lifestyle changes, including

- ➡ regular exercise (reduces mood swings and weight gain);
- ➡ sticking to a meal plan, limiting salt (to reduce bloating) and caffeine, and choosing sugar-free or low-fat treats;
- ➡ taking a multivitamin with folic acid and calcium, which in addition to keeping bones strong may ease PMS symptoms;
- ➡ taking ibuprofen to relieve headaches and cramps, and diuretics to counteract fluid retention. In cases where symptoms are severe, a class of antidepressants called serotonin reuptake inhibitors may help mood.

MENSTRUAL IRREGULARITIES

Women with diabetes, especially younger women, tend to have more irregular periods than women without diabetes. If glucose control is particularly poor, periods may stop for one or more cycles. Other menstrual irregularities include heavy bleeding, periods lasting more than six days, and cycles of more than thirty-one days. Obese women with type 2 diabetes are more likely than other women to experience menstrual irregularities, including amenorrhea, the absence of menstrual periods. Such irregularities make it difficult to chart the patterns of glucose control.

If you have diabetes and you skip a period, check with your physician to be sure you are not pregnant. Home urine-testing kits, though reliable, cannot detect pregnancy as early as a blood test ordered by your doctor.

It is possible that with the current emphasis on tight glucose control, fewer women with type 1 diabetes will experience menstrual irregularities. But women with type 1 diabetes are prone to thyroid problems, which can also cause menstrual problems.

POLYCYSTIC OVARY SYNDROME

Irregular menstrual cycles are also one of the symptoms of polycystic ovary syndrome. It is estimated that up to 27 percent of women with type 2 diabetes who are still menstruating have PCOS. Women with PCOS typically produce higher than normal levels of male hormones called androgens, resulting in excess hair growth on the face, chest, and back. Women with PCOS may also have cysts on their ovaries. Other signs of the syndrome include obesity, acne, and infertility.

PCOS is also associated with insulin resistance and a high risk of developing type 2 diabetes. Insulin resistance is particularly prevalent in women with PCOS who are also obese. Women with PCOS who don't yet have type 2 diabetes are prime candidates for lifestyle changes or medications to prevent the disease from developing.

Women who have both PCOS and diabetes can improve their menstrual cycle regularity and reduce the hairiness and acne resulting from overproduction of androgens with the same strategies that improve insulin resistance: weight loss, exercise, and medications. Additional medications and sometimes surgery might be necessary to improve fertility. The diabetes drug metformin not only controls glucose but also improves some of the abnormalities associated with PCOS. In small clinical studies metformin has been shown to increase fertility.

Both PCOS and diabetes increase the risk of cardiovascular disease, so it is critical to start prevention strategies early on. Dietary strategies for weight loss and reduction of blood pressure and lipid levels will help counter the risk of cardiovascular disease. Regular pelvic examinations and PAP smears can help catch early signs of endometrial (uterine) cancer, which women with PCOS may be at higher risk for developing. Improving the regularity of your menstrual cycle will not only help you identify any abnormal bleeding, which might be a sign of a serious problem, but also decrease your risk for uterine cancer and osteoporosis.

CONTRACEPTIVE OPTIONS

Ideally, every pregnancy for a woman with diabetes should be a planned pregnancy. It can take months of preparation to lay the groundwork for a safe pregnancy. Until then, it is extremely important to choose an effective and safe form of birth control that suits your lifestyle and personal preferences. Women with diabetes are not told to avoid any particular contraceptives, but some are considered more safe than others.

Most medical providers feel that high doses of the oral contraceptive pill ("the pill") should rarely be used, as they carry a higher risk of complications for all women, but particularly those with diabetes. Most women who take oral contraceptives are prescribed low-dose estrogen pills. Other factors particular to your health may make some contraceptives hazardous or ineffective for you. Women who smoke or have had blood clots, migraines, very high blood pressure, or certain lipid disorders, for example, are advised not to use oral contraceptives.

Below we provide a brief summary of the birth control methods

Table 5.1 Options for contraception

Method	Pros	Cons	Comments
Barrier:			
Male condom	Additional protection against sexually transmitted disease (STD)	Need to have available at time of intercourse	Most commonly used means of contraception
diaphragm	No effect on sugars	Need to insert at time of intercourse	
Intrauterine device (IUD)	No effect on sugars	Heavy periods and increase in premenstrual syndrome Infection and inflammation Requires gynecologist to insert and yearly pelvic examination to check that it remains in place	Recommendation on a case-by-case basis
Oral contraceptive pill	Relatively easy to use Comes in patch form	No protection against STDs Possible effect on sugars Increases risk of heart disease if high risk to begin with Risk of blood clots	Good for women with no preexisting risk for heart disease or blood clots
Depo-Provera	Easy to use	Injection every three months Risk of osteoporosis (thinning of the bones) Weight gain	
Tubal ligation	Single procedure	Permanent	For women who have completed child bearing or are at high risk for pregnancy-related complications

currently available in the United States (see also Table 5.1). The failure rates come from the Food and Drug Administration and are based on clinical trials submitted to the FDA before the products were approved. The failure rates include pregnancies related to missed doses. For example, if you take an oral contraceptive and never miss a dose, failure rates may be even lower than those listed. We have no reason to believe that the effectiveness or safety of these methods is different for women with diabetes.

Remember that it is still possible to get pregnant in your forties and even early fifties—the years before menopause, when your periods become more irregular. If you do not want to get pregnant, use birth control until your periods have stopped for more than a year.

HORMONAL METHODS

ORAL CONTRACEPTIVES—COMBINED PILL (MANY DIFFERENT BRAND NAMES). The pill has been around for more than forty years and is the most popular form of birth control in the United States. It blocks ovulation through the combined actions of estrogen and progestin (an artificial form of progesterone). The doses of estrogen in the pill are generally lower now than in the past and are a safe and effective means of birth control. The pill is taken daily and is now available in a chewable tablet. The failure rate is one to two pregnancies for every one hundred women taking it. An added advantage of the oral contraceptive pill is that it reduces the risk of ovarian and uterine cancer up to 50 percent regardless of how long you take it. It can also help decrease premenstrual syndrome, protect against pelvic inflammatory disease, and possibly increase bone density. Side effects include headache, weight gain, acne, and depression, depending on the formulation. Most lower-dose pills are well tolerated.

> *The male condom is the only contraceptive method that offers adequate protection against sexually transmitted diseases, and even it is not foolproof.*

ORAL NINETY-ONE-DAY REGIMEN (BRAND NAME: SEASONALE). The ninety-one-day regimen consists of a daily pill with both estrogen and progestin that results in only one menstrual period every three months (twelve weeks of active pills followed by one week of inactive pills, during which menstruation occurs). The failure rate is one to two women per one hundred. Many women prefer this form of oral contraceptive to the traditional combination pill.

ORAL PROGESTIN-ONLY MINIPILL (BRAND NAMES: MI-CRONOR, OVRETTE, NOR-QD). The progestin-only pill (or POP) acts on mucus in the cervix to prevent sperm from reaching the egg. It is taken daily and has a failure rate of two pregnancies for every one hundred women taking it. This pill is the preferred option for women with diabetes who have other medical problems, such as high cholesterol and high blood pressure. It can also be used during breastfeeding, as it does not suppress milk production. The problem with this class of pills is that because they contain only progesterone, there is an increased risk of breakthrough menstrual bleeding (bleeding between menstrual cycles). If you experience intercyclical bleeding, you should use a back-up means of birth control such as a condom.

PATCH (BRAND NAME: ORTHO EVRA). The patch is a new delivery system for hormonal birth control. A skin patch worn on the lower abdomen, buttocks, or upper body releases estrogen and progestin, which are then absorbed into the bloodstream. The patch is worn for three weeks (replaced with a new patch each week), followed by one week with no patch, during which menstruation occurs. The failure rate is one to two per one hundred women, though it appears to be less effective in women who weigh more than 198 pounds.

VAGINAL CONTRACEPTIVE RING (BRAND NAME: NUVA-RING). The vaginal ring is inserted into the vagina by the woman. It then releases estrogen and progestin. The ring remains in place for three weeks and is removed for one week, during which menstruation occurs. The failure rate is one to two per one hundred women.

INJECTION (BRAND NAME: DEPO-PROVERA). Depo-Provera shots are injections of progestin given once every three months. The progestin acts by inhibiting ovulation, preventing sperm from reaching the egg, and preventing a fertilized egg from implanting in the uterus. The failure rate is less than one per one hundred women.

It can cause weight gain, mood changes, and increase the risk of osteo-porosis with long-term use. Depo shots are usually given by a health care provider.

INJECTION (BRAND NAME: LUNELLE). Lunelle is a once-monthly shot of progestin and estrogen. As with Depo-Provera, these injections must be given by a health care professional. The failure rate is less than one per one hundred women.

BARRIER METHODS

MALE CONDOMS. The male condom is a thin sheath that is placed over an erect penis to contain the sperm after ejaculation. It is used once and discarded. Most condoms are made of either latex rubber or polyurethane, which is less likely than latex to cause an allergic reaction. Condoms are the best protection against sexually transmitted diseases, though those made from natural materials (such as those labeled "lambskin," made from lamb intestines) are not as effective as synthetic condoms at preventing disease and have a higher risk of breakage. The failure rate is eleven out of one hundred women.

FEMALE CONDOMS. The female condom is a polyurethane sheath shaped like the male condom; the closed end has a flexible ring and is inserted into the vagina, while the open end remains outside, partially covering the labia, the outer lips of the vagina. It is used once and discarded. Unlike the male condom, it does not offer reliable protection against sexually transmitted diseases, and it has a high failure rate of twenty-one out of one hundred women.

DIAPHRAGM WITH SPERMICIDE. The diaphragm is a dome-shaped rubber disk with a flexible rim, which allows a woman to fold it in half to insert it up against the cervix. It acts by blocking the sperm from reaching the uterus. A spermicide—a sperm-killing gel or cream—is inserted into the disk before it is placed in the vagina. The diaphragm should be left in place at least six hours (and no more than twenty-four hours) after sex (additional spermicide should be inserted into the vagina if intercourse is repeated). The failure rate is seventeen out of one hundred women.

CERVICAL CAP WITH SPERMICIDE. The cervical cap is similar to the diaphragm, but it can stay in place for forty-eight hours and protects during repeated intercourse. The failure rate is seventeen to twenty-three out of one hundred women.

CONTRACEPTIVE SPONGE. The soft, disk-shaped synthetic sponge containing spermicide is inserted into the vagina to cover the cervix. It protects against pregnancy for twenty-four hours and should be kept in for at least six to eight hours. The sponge was taken off the market in 1995, not because of safety concerns, but because the manufacturer decided that it would be too costly to fix problems in the production process. This contraceptive device, which is available without a prescription, was reapproved by the FDA to return to the market in April 2005. The failure rate is eighteen to twenty-eight per one hundred women. Studies suggest that it may be more effective for women who have never delivered a baby.

INTRAUTERINE DEVICE

IUD (BRAND NAMES: PARAGARD T, MIRENA). The IUD is a device inserted into the uterus by a health care professional. It works by preventing the sperm and egg from meeting or by inhibiting implantation. At one time IUDs were not recommended for women with diabetes because of the risk of pelvic inflammatory disease (an infection of the reproductive tract), but today's IUDs are much safer. Depending on the type of IUD, the device can be left in place for one to ten years. It may cause increased menstrual bleeding or cramping, especially in women who have never been pregnant. The failure rate is less than one out of one hundred women.

STERILIZATION

FEMALE STERILIZATION. Various surgical techniques are used to block the fallopian tubes so the egg can't travel to the uterus and get fertilized. The failure rate is less than one per one hundred women. The procedure is considered permanent but may be reversed with surgery.

MALE STERILIZATION. The vasectomy is a quick outpatient surgical procedure in which the vas deferens is cut or tied so that sperm can't travel from the testicles to the penis. The failure rate is less than one pregnancy per one hundred women. The procedure is considered permanent but may be reversed with surgery.

EMERGENCY CONTRACEPTION

POST-COITAL "EMERGENCY" CONTRACEPTIVE ("PLAN B"). Emergency contraception consists of a pill containing a relatively large dose of progestin that must be taken within seventy-two hours of unprotected sex, and a second tablet that is taken twelve hours after the first. This form of contraception is currently available only by prescription, though in some states a pharmacist can dispense it. Plan B can reduce the risk of pregnancy by 90 percent if used promptly within seventy-two hours of intercourse. It is used only for emergency situations, such as when a condom breaks mid-cycle, and is not a regular means of birth control.

PLANNING FOR PREGNANCY

Deciding to have a baby is a private decision, but preparing to have one should involve your health care team. In contrast to the not-too-distant past, when birth defects and miscarriage were common, nowadays a woman with diabetes who keeps her blood glucose levels near normal

POSSIBLE COMPLICATIONS OF POORLY CONTROLLED DIABETES IN PREGNANCY

Baby

- Increased risk of miscarriage
- Fetal birth defects of heart, spine, or gastrointestinal and urinary tracts
- Low blood sugar
- Macrosomia (larger-than-normal baby, which increases the risk of birth trauma and need for cesarean section)
- Premature labor
- Stillbirth

Mother

- Worsening glucose control
- Increased risk of diabetic ketoacidosis
- High blood pressure and preeclampsia/eclampsia (toxemia)
- Progression of preexisting eye and kidney disease
- Urinary tract and kidney infections

These complications are the incentive to get your blood glucose levels under control before and during pregnancy. Doing so will significantly reduce the risk of problems for you and your baby.

both before and during pregnancy has almost the same chance of delivering a healthy baby as a woman without diabetes.

To maximize your chances of having a healthy pregnancy and a healthy baby, though, you must involve your health care team *before* you stop using contraceptives. The team includes your diabetes physician, a dietitian, and a diabetes nurse educator. Many women with diabetes, especially type 1 diabetes, may be referred to an obstetrician who specializes in high-risk pregnancies, either before or after they become pregnant.

Controlling glucose before and during pregnancy is particularly important because high levels of blood sugar and other metabolic substances can pass through the placenta to the baby and affect its early organ development. Malformations in the heart, urinary tract, digestive tract, and spinal cord can result. Most organs form in the first six to eight weeks of pregnancy, usually before many women even know they are pregnant. Thus, maintaining tight control of glucose as you prepare for pregnancy will provide the best environment for your developing baby. This is true regardless of the type of diabetes you have.

Fortunately, intensive control of diabetes is now recommended as part of routine diabetes care, so more women than ever are prepared for pregnancy.

THE 7 PERCENT SOLUTION

Before you become pregnant, your goal should be to achieve a hemoglobin A_{1c} that is no greater than 1 percent above the normal range. Recall that this is the blood test that reflects the status of your glucose levels for the previous two to three months. A score of 4 percent to 6 percent is normal for people without diabetes. The goal of diabetes care is to keep your score at less than 7 percent, and this is also the goal before you become pregnant. Above that percentage, the incidence of birth defects rises.

To achieve these levels before conception, you should aim for the following plasma glucose readings:

- ➡ Before meals: 80–120 mg/dl (4.4–6.6 mmol/l).
- ➡ Two hours after meals: under 180 mg/dl (under 10 mmol/l).

Women with type 1 diabetes will need to practice intensive insulin therapy to maintain these near-normal glucose levels. They should have had lots of practice, since intensive therapy is now the standard of care. The sugar goals are even more stringent during pregnancy, however, so be prepared to step up your efforts. You will need to check your blood sugar levels even more frequently—six to eight or even more times a day—and make precise adjustments to the dosages and frequency of insulin you give yourself.

Women with type 2 diabetes who are planning a pregnancy may

COMMON MEDICATIONS SAFE IN PREGNANCY

Acetominophen (Tylenol)

Ibuprofen (Motrin, Advil)

Salicylates (aspirin)

Insulins

Beta blockers

Thyroid medications

Famotidine (Pepcid)

have to switch to insulin therapy to get tighter control of their glucose levels if dietary efforts do not suffice. The switch from oral medications to insulin will probably be done anyway once you get pregnant, since none of the oral antidiabetic drugs currently prescribed have been approved for use during pregnancy.

If you have type 1 or type 2 diabetes and are contemplating pregnancy, you should have a thorough physical examination. Your doctor will assess any new or existing diabetic complications and evaluate heart and thyroid function. She will also review any medications you take to ensure that they are safe during pregnancy. ACE inhibitors taken for high blood pressure and cholesterol-lowering medications, for example, have to be discontinued during pregnancy. Other, safer medications such as beta blockers can be taken in their place.

You will also be started on prenatal vitamins and folic acid supplements. Women with diabetes need more folic acid than is found in a regular multivitamin because their babies are at higher risk for spina bifida, a defect in the early development and formation of the spinal cord (prenatal vitamins have sufficient folic acid). Anyone who smokes cigarettes will be strongly advised to quit and shown ways to do it.

Preparing for pregnancy may take three to six months. You'll want to be certain that you have adjusted your diabetes regimen sufficiently to achieve good blood sugar levels and that the hemoglobin A_{1c} reflects acceptable control. Your physician will give you the green light to start trying to conceive. At that point you can stop using birth control.

Fertility problems and miscarriage used to be common for women with type 1 diabetes, but the good news is that with careful control of blood sugar levels, this is no longer true. Women with PCOS and type 2 diabetes may have trouble getting pregnant, however. This problem can often be resolved once the PCOS is treated. Anyone having difficulties getting pregnant after six months of unprotected intercourse should consult her physician.

WILL MY BABY GET DIABETES?

There is no way to know for sure if your baby will develop diabetes. Many poorly understood variables underlie the inheritance and development of diabetes. Many children or adults get either type 1 or type 2 diabetes even when no one in their family has ever had the disease. But both forms are inherited, and having a first-degree relative (parent, child, or sibling) with diabetes increases someone's chances of getting it. Environmental factors such as diet, lifestyle, and infections may also trigger the disease in those who are susceptible.

Interestingly, studies have shown that children are more likely to get type 1 diabetes if their father has type 1 diabetes than if their mother has it. Remember that type 1 diabetes is relatively rare in the general population, affecting no more than one of every two hundred individuals over a lifetime. If the father has diabetes, the chance that his child will also develop type 1 diabetes is about 6 percent; if you are a woman with type 1 diabetes, the chance is about 3–5 percent that your child will develop type 1 diabetes.

As part of the preparation for pregnancy, all women with diabetes should receive counseling on their family's constellation of risk factors. Genetic susceptibility to the disease is usually not a reason to avoid pregnancy.

DIABETES AND PREGNANCY: WHAT IS YOUR RISK?

One of the grand moments in life, when you're ready for it, is to find out that you're pregnant. That moment and the months to come are a time of excitement and nervous anticipation. But on top of all the regular concerns about a healthy pregnancy, a pregnant woman with diabetes must also contend with the additional challenges of living with a chronic disease. It takes extra work to keep mother and child safe. But a healthy baby is worth the effort.

Pregnancy can worsen the complications of diabetes, including retinopathy (eye disease), nephropathy (kidney disease), and neuropathy (nerve disease). But pregnancy does not appear to increase a woman's risk of developing these complications permanently. If diabetic complications do worsen during pregnancy, they often return to their prepregnancy state after delivery. The appropriate medical specialists should follow up on any existing complications throughout the pregnancy. For example, you will need to see your eye doctor more frequently during your pregnancy. Blood pressure, which tends to run high in women with type 1 and type 2 diabetes, will be closely monitored throughout the pregnancy.

TREATMENT DURING PREGNANCY

In an ideal world, you would have planned for your pregnancy as described above. But if not, the important thing is to see your physician immediately. Your health care team will determine the frequency of appointments, as well as who you need to see and when. If your blood sugar levels are not in an acceptable range, you will need to adjust your therapy as soon as possible. Your level of physical activity and diabetes medications will also be reassessed. Most women can continue the same level of exercise as before pregnancy, but you should avoid activities that increase the risk of injury. You should also keep your pulse less than 140 beats per minute.

Most of what we know about diabetes during pregnancy is based on the experiences of women with type 1. But as the number of women of childbearing age with type 2 diabetes has increased steadily, so has the number of pregnant women with type 2. We now know that type 2 diabetes poses just as much risk to mother and child as does type 1.

WOMEN WITH TYPE 1 DIABETES

If your blood sugars are not considered acceptable, you will have to start intensive therapy or make adjustments to your current therapy. Because of the increased risk for fetal malformations, if your HgbA$_{1c}$ is high at the time of conception your doctor might talk about the risks of continuing the pregnancy.

In the quest to bring glucose levels as close to normal as possible, you may find that they sometimes slip down too low. Episodes of hypoglycemia typically increase during pregnancy. To be safe, you should always carry hard candy and glucose tablets for those times when your blood sugar is too low. Make sure your family and friends know the symptoms of hypoglycemia, too: nervousness, perspiration, shakiness, light-headedness, sleepiness, confusion, and difficulty speaking (see Chapter 4).

Women following intensive therapy for years may be particularly susceptible to "hypoglycemia unawareness": not recognizing symptoms and therefore not being able to treat hypoglycemia quickly. Any episode of severe hypoglycemia can decrease the warning symptoms of subsequent hypoglycemia and make another episode more likely. Your health care team can help you adjust your regimen to decrease these episodes, but the stringent goals of therapy during pregnancy do make hypoglycemia more common. Even though the placenta protects the baby from low blood sugars, hypoglycemia is still dangerous for the mother if allowed to become severe, with possible confusion, loss of consciousness, or seizures.

Table 5.2   Glucose goals during pregnancy

	Fasting and before meals	1 hour after eating	A$_{1c}$	Comments
Prior to conception	80–120	100–155	<7 percent; normal if possible	Avoid severe low blood sugars
During pregnancy (for those with pre-existing diabetes)	60–100	100–140	<7 percent; normal if possible	Check for ketones as directed by your medical care team
Gestational diabetes	<100	<130		May need insulin during pregnancy if sugars not well controlled

Note: To stay in the targeted range, some women need to test their blood glucose levels seven to eight times a day or more and make insulin adjustments.

Women with type 1 diabetes should also be on alert for ketoacidosis, a condition that develops when glucose levels rise too high (see Chapter 4). The glucose level that spirals the body into diabetic ketoacidosis is lower during pregnancy than it would be otherwise. (See Table 5.2 for glucose goals during pregnancy.)

Pregnancy represents a dynamic state with different challenges at different stages. During the first trimester (month one to three), morning nausea may decrease your dietary intake or make it erratic, further complicating your blood sugar control. During the last trimester, insulin requirements often increase dramatically, to the extent that women frequently need to double their doses to maintain acceptable glucose control. Diabetes also increases the risk of preterm labor or preeclampsia (which can prevent the placenta from getting enough blood), which may require bedrest.

As we have discussed, early control of blood sugar is key to preventing fetal malformations. Control of blood sugar levels during the rest of the pregnancy is required to prevent your baby from growing too large (a condition called macrosomia). If blood sugars are not tightly controlled, a "large for date" baby results, often complicating delivery. A cesarean section, whereby the baby is surgically delivered, or a premature delivery may be required to lower the risk of birth trauma and injury. In addition, the newborns may suffer from low blood sugar and respiratory and other problems, necessitating close monitoring and in some cases medical observation in a neonatal intensive care unit. All these problems can be prevented, or at least reduced, with tight glucose control throughout your pregnancy.

WOMEN WITH TYPE 2 DIABETES

Women whose diabetes has been managed by diet alone may continue this way as long as their blood sugar levels are considered acceptable. Those who are on diabetes medications will be switched to insulin, as this is the only diabetes medication currently approved for use during pregnancy. Most women can return to their prepregnancy medication regimen following delivery.

Your weight gain will also be monitored. If you start out overweight, your doctor may recommend that you gain no more than fifteen to twenty-five pounds, if not less. You won't want to gain more than is necessary for a healthy baby, but you do need to be sure you are getting all the nutrients you need.

Some women who are very obese (defined as a BMI of 40 or greater; see Appendix 1) may not need to gain any weight. The state of obesity itself can lead to complications during pregnancy, such as high blood pressure, prolonged delivery, and a greater chance of cesarean delivery.

Women who begin pregnancy in the normal weight range can expect to gain about twenty-two to twenty-seven pounds.

DIAGNOSING GESTATIONAL DIABETES (GDM)

Between 3 and 5 percent of all women develop diabetes during pregnancy. Gestational diabetes is defined as high glucose levels that are first recognized during pregnancy. Because GDM is not diagnosed until late in pregnancy, the fetal malformations that can affect the babies of women with prepregnancy diabetes are not a concern with gestational diabetes. Women with GDM are at risk for producing extra-large babies, though, which can present problems during delivery. Therefore, tight glucose targets are also necessary in cases of gestational diabetes.

For many women with GDM, dietary changes will usually keep blood sugars in an acceptable range. Unless there is a medical reason against it, women with GDM should be able to engage in moderate exercise. Insulin is necessary, however, for those who cannot achieve targeted glucose levels through changes in diet and activity level.

All pregnant women (except those considered at low risk) should be screened for gestational diabetes between their twenty-fourth and twenty-eighth week of pregnancy. Those at high risk (essentially the same risk factors noted in Chapter 2 for type 2 diabetes) should be screened earlier in their pregnancy and retested between weeks twenty-four and twenty-eight. Women with any of the following risk factors should be screened for GDM:

→ above age twenty-five
→ above ideal body weight
→ first-degree relative with diabetes (sister, mother, father)
→ member of high-risk ethnic group (Hispanic, African American, Asian American, Pacific Islander, Native American)
→ history of glucose intolerance
→ previous large baby (more than nine pounds)

After the first five to six months of pregnancy, a woman's need for insulin increases. As the placenta grows, it secretes hormones that counteract the effects of the insulin. In most women, insulin secretion increases to meet this demand and blood sugars remain normal. However, in women who are predisposed to diabetes, insulin levels don't keep up with the increased demand and blood sugars rise.

Usually glucose levels return to normal shortly after the birth of

Table 5.3 Oral glucose tolerance test scores to diagnose gestational diabetes

Plasma glucose (mg/dL)	50-gram screening test	100-gram diagnostic test
Fasting	—	95–105
1 hour	140	180–190
2 hour	—	155–165
3 hour	—	140–145

Note: Women who score 140 or greater on the 50-gram test take the 100-gram diagnostic test. A diagnosis of gestational diabetes is made if two or more readings (fasting, 1 hour, 2 hour, or 3 hour) fall into the ranges shown above.

Source: Adapted from the American Diabetes Association (Position Statement). Standards of Medical Care for Patients with Diabetes. *Diabetes Care,* 29 (Supplement 1) (2006): S6.

the baby. But women who have had gestational diabetes are at greatly increased risk of developing diabetes later on, either with their next pregnancy or often within five to ten years after being diagnosed with GDM.

The oral glucose tolerance test (OGTT) is used to screen for and diagnose gestational diabetes, which almost always has no symptoms. A preliminary step is usually taken to weed out women with normal glucose levels. Women are given fifty grams of a sugary syrup to drink, then after an hour their glucose levels are measured. Those whose levels are greater than 140 mg/dl (some say the cut-off should be 130 mg/dl) then go on to a more definitive, three-hour diagnostic test (see Table 5.3).

In the more definitive diagnostic test, a fasting glucose test is performed. The woman then drinks one hundred grams of the sugary syrup. Her blood glucose levels are then checked three more times over the next three hours (after one hour, after two hours, and after three hours). If at least two of the blood sugar levels are above the normal range, she is diagnosed with gestational diabetes.

Pregnant women are already anxious about their babies, so it can be particularly frightening to be diagnosed with gestational diabetes. The babies of women with GDM, like those of women with type 1 and type 2 diabetes, tend to be bigger than average. But in general, with good care, both mother and baby do fine.

Most women find that their glucose tolerance returns to normal after delivery. Glucose tolerance should be tested using the nonpregnancy screening strategy (see Chapter 2) six to twelve weeks after delivery, either by an obstetrician or by a primary care provider, when most women's glucose levels have returned to normal.

Between 30 and 50 percent of women with GDM will develop type 2 diabetes in the five years after they are diagnosed with GDM, especially those who are already at high risk for diabetes. Obesity, the need for insulin during the pregnancy, and repeated episodes of GDM all increase the risk of future diabetes. So it is important to repeat the OGTT test every one to three years thereafter. Consider your GDM a crystal ball for a future that doesn't have to happen. See Chapter 3 for strategies to prevent type 2 diabetes.

If you had gestational diabetes, you should alert your child's physician. Your child may be at greater risk for obesity and insulin resistance, especially during adolescence.

EATING FOR TWO

When you are pregnant, it's more important than ever not to skip meals or snacks. You'll need more calories during pregnancy to support a growing baby, and your dietitian or diabetes nurse educator will adapt your meal plan to meet these demands. Women who are overweight or obese may be able to use their extra stores of calories to supply some of this demand.

If you are experiencing morning sickness, you may also have to modify your meal plan by eating smaller, more frequent meals. Sometimes eating crackers or pretzels when you get up in the morning helps. Women with type 1, type 2, or gestational diabetes will receive individualized plans for nutrition therapy. But here are some general guidelines:

➡ Since carbohydrates have the greatest impact on blood glucose levels, try to keep the amount you eat consistent at each meal from day to day (see the section on carbohydrates in Chapter 7).

➡ Eat a variety of foods to get the nutrients you need, particularly whole-grain breads, fruits, vegetables, iron-rich foods (lean meat, poultry, fish, leafy green vegetables), and calcium-rich foods (dairy products, some nuts, and green vegetables).

➡ Take a daily prenatal vitamin.

➡ Avoid alcohol altogether and limit caffeine to less than 2 caffeinated drinks per day (coffee, tea, caffeinated soda, and chocolate; remember, one chocolate bar is equal to one-quarter cup of coffee).

➡ Use only artificial sweeteners that have been approved for use during pregnancy: aspartame, acesulfame-K, and sucralose (saccharin is strongly discouraged). (See Table 3.3.)

➡ Do not use "eating for two" as an excuse to overindulge. Weight gain is expected for most pregnancies but is not required for those who are overweight or obese.

LABOR AND DELIVERY

Many women with well-controlled type 1 and type 2 diabetes carry their babies to full term without any problems. If the developing baby is large, however, the obstetrician may decide to induce labor a little early—often after thirty-five weeks, as soon as the baby's lungs have matured—rather than wait the full forty weeks. In such cases, the doctor will administer a drug that triggers the birth process. Babies of women with diabetes are commonly on the large side, because the baby reacts to high levels of maternal glucose by producing excess insulin, which acts as a growth hormone. Sometimes the baby gets too big to be delivered vaginally and the obstetrician must perform a cesarean section.

Labor is like a form of exercise and has a glucose-lowering effect. Because your body is working so hard and using a great deal of glucose as energy, you may not need insulin by the time you are in active labor. The glucose levels of all women with diabetes will be carefully monitored throughout labor and delivery.

Women with type 1 diabetes often find that their insulin needs decrease the first few weeks after delivery. Others with type 1 experience fluctuations in their glucose levels. You will need to check your blood sugar levels frequently to avoid complications that might interfere with your ability to care for your baby properly.

Women with type 2 diabetes who began insulin during pregnancy may not need to take it after delivery. Oral agents must be used with caution, however, since some of them appear in breast milk and should not be taken if a woman is nursing.

All new mothers are exhausted and overwhelmed by the new demands placed on them. Though your new world revolves around the baby, you have to remember that to take good care of your baby, you first have to take good care of yourself.

TO NURSE OR NOT TO NURSE

Study after study demonstrates the benefits of breastfeeding. Mother's milk is an ideal source of nutrition for most infants and provides health benefits for both mother and baby. There is strong evidence, for example, that mother's milk decreases the incidence or severity of diarrheal diseases, ear infections, respiratory infections, and urinary tract infections, among other illnesses in the newborn. Women who breastfeed return to their prepregnancy weight more quickly than other women and have reduced incidences of ovarian cancer and, at least before menopause, of breast cancer. Breastfeeding is also a wonderful bonding experience between mother and baby.

As long as your physician doesn't identify a medical reason you shouldn't breastfeed (a medication you are taking, for example), the choice is up to you. Many of the medications for diabetes are safe during breastfeeding, including insulin and many of the sulfonyureas and acarbose. We don't have enough evidence yet to know about the safety of metformin and the thiazolidinediones. Review your treatment plan with your medical provider to see if the medications you are taking are safe during breastfeeding.

Some women with diabetes have a hard time getting their milk supply started. This is particularly true if for some reason the baby needed to be separated from the mother to be treated in an intensive-care nursery. In the days when near-normal blood sugars were not the norm, women with type 1 diabetes were more prone to breast infections while trying to nurse. But most women who decide to breastfeed are able to do so successfully.

Women who breastfeed require additional calories, so meal plans should be adjusted accordingly. A snack as well as drinking water or a caffeine-free drink are usually recommended before or during nursing. Dosages of insulin or other diabetes medications will also be adjusted on the basis of your new level of activity so that you can maintain good blood glucose control. You might prepare a box of supplies to bring with you wherever you nurse, including water, hard candies, glucose test strips, and your meter. Remember, the insulin you take works on you, not the baby.

Breastfeeding adds another dimension to the challenge of managing the care of a new infant as well as your own care. But the payoff is unquestionable.

MENOPAUSE MATTERS

At the other end of a woman's reproductive life—in no way signaling the end of life—is menopause. A woman has entered menopause when she has not had a menstrual period for one year. Before that time, there is a gradual slowdown in the production of estrogen and progesterone for about five to ten years, a phase of life called perimenopause. Ovulation begins to decrease during this time, so not all cycles involve the release of an egg. The average age for menopause is fifty-one, but it can occur anytime between ages forty-two and fifty-eight. Some women with type 1 diabetes are prone to early ovarian failure, another manifestation of autoimmunity, which results in early menopause (younger than age forty-two).

The levels of the female hormones estrogen and progesterone fluctuate erratically during perimenopause until the ovaries stop producing them altogether. The fluctuations in these hormones can cause hot flashes, vaginal dryness, and mood changes. Women with diabetes may find that their blood glucose levels also fluctuate during this period and become harder to control. They then level out after menopause. Hot flashes and night sweats make it more difficult to sense hypoglycemia, since the symptoms are similar.

Women with diabetes are prone to yeast infections and urinary tract infections (we'll talk more about both later in this chapter), which are more common for all women as they enter menopause. These infections may increase as a result of the drying effect of estrogen loss on the vaginal mucous membranes and changes in bladder function. Women also tend to gain weight at this time of life—particularly around the waist and abdomen. Their lipid profiles—the amount of "good" and "bad" cholesterol and triglycerides—change too as estrogen is reduced, in a way that is less heart-protective. The rate of bone loss increases at menopause.

Many women find that at menopause they need to adjust their dosages of insulin or other diabetes medications as well as their diet and level of physical activity. There are dietary strategies to counter the effects of menopause: soy for hot flashes, for example, and calcium supplements (and exercise with weights) for bone loss. Now that the risk of cardiovascular disease is even greater, women should be evaluated for additional ways to reduce this risk, perhaps by taking a cholesterol-lowering drug.

HORMONE (ESTROGEN) REPLACEMENT THERAPY (HRT)

At one time it was almost routine to counteract the symptoms of menopause with the use of hormone replacement therapy. It was also thought that HRT helped prevent heart disease and osteoporosis, a disease in which the bones become less dense and susceptible to breaking. By the year 2000, about 40 percent of all menopausal women, including women with diabetes, were taking estrogen in the form of pills, patches, or vaginal creams. But with the published results of the

Women's Health Initiative study in 2002—which showed a 30 percent increase in heart disease in women on hormone replacement therapy and evidence that HRT increased the risk of breast and uterine cancer—physicians did an about-face. The risks of HRT now appear to outweigh its benefits. HRT is now recommended only as a short-term treatment at the lowest dose possible to relieve hot flashes and vaginal atrophy (thinning of vaginal wall tissue).

The jury stayed out a bit longer on whether HRT should still be recommended for women with diabetes. Some studies had suggested that women on HRT have better blood glucose control than those not on it. But the balance now appears to be tipped against using HRT for women with diabetes too, unless absolutely necessary. Women with diabetes are already at increased risk of heart disease, so any drug that causes further risk should be stopped.

COMMON CONDITIONS AFFECTING WOMEN

Several infections or diseases common among women affect those with diabetes even more. High levels of sugar in the bladder and vaginal fluid, for example, provide a ripe environment for yeast infections and urinary tract infections, common for young sexually active women and those in menopause. Be mindful of these possibilities so a physician can help you get relief.

YEAST INFECTIONS (ONE TYPE OF VAGINAL INFECTION)

Extremely common, yeast infections cause severe itching or burning in the vagina and a thick, cottage cheese–like discharge. A health care provider should diagnose a first-time infection to rule out other vaginal infections or sexually transmitted diseases. Over-the-counter treatments are available for those who have recurring episodes of infection.

But see a physician if you are pregnant or if nonprescription treatments, such as antifungal suppositories or creams, do not work; oral therapy such as Diflucan can be prescribed. For some women, chronic yeast infections are a symptom of diabetes.

VAGINITIS (VAGINAL INFLAMMATIONS IN GENERAL)

Vaginitis is an inflammation of the vagina caused by various organisms or by the low level of estrogen that occurs after menopause. A health care provider makes the diagnosis based on the appearance of the vaginal discharge (white, cottage cheesy, green, or frothy, for example), the symptoms of burning and itching, and the results of cultures taken and tested.

URINARY TRACT INFECTIONS

Infections of the urinary tract occur when bacteria grow somewhere in the urinary system, including the urethra (the canal through which urine is released from the bladder), the bladder, the kidneys, or the ureter (the tube that carries urine to the bladder). Internal pain during urination may be the only symptom, though some women feel an urgency to urinate though just a little urine comes out. Urinary tract infections can be more difficult to treat in women with diabetes; and, for some women, chronic recurrent urinary tract infections can be a sign of diabetes. Women with diabetes whose urinary tract infections go untreated also have a higher risk of kidney infection (pyelonephritis), a potentially serious complication.

URINARY INCONTINENCE

Women in general are at risk of urinary incontinence (loss of bladder control) as they age, and diabetes adds to that risk. Women with diabetes are particularly susceptible to "urge incontinence," the sudden, un-

The urinary tract

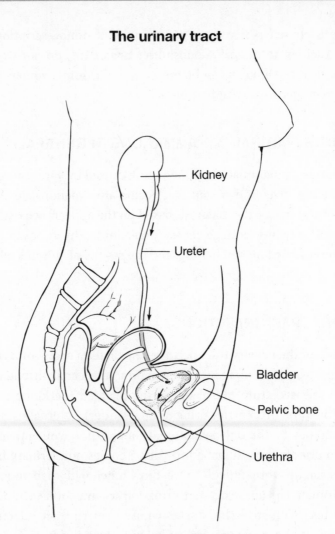

Urine is produced in the kidneys and flows to the bladder through the ureters before exiting through the urethra.

For some women, chronic urinary tract infections can be a sign of diabetes. (K. J. Carlson, S. A. Eisenstat, and T. Ziporyn, *The New Harvard Guide to Women's Health* [Cambridge, Mass.: Harvard University Press, 2004], p. 302.)

controllable urge to urinate. "Stress incontinence" is loss of urine after a physical activity such as exercise, coughing, sneezing, or laughing. Childbirth, aging, and obesity are common risk factors for this condition.

Urinary incontinence that is specific to women with diabetes is probably related to a form of neuropathy (nerve damage) that affects the bladder. What appears to happen is that decreased sensory signals from the bladder result in the distention of the bladder over time. As the bladder stretches, it loses elasticity. Before long, the ability to empty the bladder effectively is lost. A big, urine-filled bladder is more prone to leaking, and stress incontinence occurs. Urinary tract infections are also common with bladder distention.

One strategy to treat this problem is to urinate frequently "by the clock." In other words, don't wait until you feel the urge to urinate. Try to empty your bladder on a regular schedule—at least every three to four hours or less—whether you feel the need to go or not. You can help empty your bladder by pushing down with your fingertips over the bladder (located in the lower abdomen) as you urinate. Intensive blood glucose control and weight loss are being scrutinized as ways to prevent urinary incontinence or to reduce its severity. Medication or surgery can help in severe cases.

THYROID DISEASE

The thyroid is a small gland in the neck responsible for producing the hormones that control the body's metabolism, the process of converting foods and oxygen into energy. Up to 20 percent of women with type 1 diabetes have either an overactive (Graves' disease) or an underactive thyroid, conditions that are much more prevalent in women than in men. Thyroid disorders, particularly hypothyroidism (underactive thyroid), appear to be more common in women with type 2 diabetes. Thyroid problems are also prevalent right after childbirth.

Thyroid dysfunction can affect glucose control and make lipid abnormalities worse, a major risk factor for cardiovascular disease. Symptoms of an overactive thyroid include otherwise unexplained weight loss, fatigue, nervousness, a fast heart rate or palpitations, tremors, hair loss, nails breaking, irregular periods, and feeling warm even when it's cold. Hypothyroidism—an underactive thyroid—has almost the opposite symptoms: weight gain, feeling sluggish and cold, constipation, and a slow heart rate. All these symptoms are nonspecific and can be very subtle, so women with diabetes should be screened regularly for thyroid abnormalities, whether or not they have symptoms. A simple blood test should be done every one to three years for women with type 1, and at diagnosis and every five years thereafter for those with type 2.

OSTEOPOROSIS

Studies have demonstrated a reduction in bone mineral density in women with type 1 diabetes, particularly after menopause. This condition may be linked to poor diabetes control. Low bone mass is called osteopenia and, if more severe, osteoporosis, a disease in which bones (such as the hips) are vulnerable to fractures or, in the case of the spine, to curvature, leading to a stooped posture. Women with type 2 diabetes who are overweight may, in fact, have high bone density, which may be protective. Nonetheless, there is some evidence that they also have a greater risk for certain types of fractures after menopause, particularly of the foot and the hip. This susceptibility may be due at least in part to the increased risk of falling associated with diabetic neuropathy and retinopathy.

The optimal time for routine screening of bone density is still being debated, but most experts agree that you should have a bone-density screening at the start of menopause and every one to two years thereafter. Given that women actually begin losing bone mass at age thirty-five, these recommendations will probably change as more research is done.

ENDOMETRIAL CANCER

There is no definitive link between diabetes and particular cancers, but we do know that being overweight or obese in general increases a woman's risk of cancer. Obesity is a major risk factor for endometrial cancer, as well as for the precancerous condition hyperplasia, a thickening of the lining of the uterus. Obesity may explain the connection between endometrial cancer and type 2 diabetes. PCOS is another risk factor for uterine cancer, and it too is associated with type 2 diabetes. In any case, abnormal menstrual bleeding during perimenopause can be an early symptom of hyperplasia or endometrial cancer. This kind of cancer is usually curable if detected at an early stage. If you notice that your periods are becoming increasingly irregular, ask your health care provider if further evaluation is indicated.

> There is no definitive link between diabetes and particular cancers, but we do know that being overweight or obese in general increases a woman's risk of cancer.

SEXUAL HEALTH

Sexual function in women is a quintessential example of how delicately interwoven are the physical and emotional aspects of health. Women's sexual problems are more subtle than men's and difficult to quantify scientifically. Diabetes is the most common cause of erectile dysfunction or impotence in men, attributed largely to complications of diabetes like neuropathy and vascular disease. Though we now know that some women with diabetes also experience sexual difficulties, we don't know why.

The main problem that women with diabetes report more frequently than women without diabetes is vaginal dryness. Lubrication of the vagina, like erection of the penis, is a vascular response to sexual arousal. If the vagina remains dry, sexual intercourse can be painful

MEDICATIONS THAT CAUSE VAGINAL DRYNESS
Allergy medications such as antihistamines
Certain ulcer, blood pressure, and antidepressant medications
Tamoxifen (used to treat breast cancer)

and an orgasm less likely. Vaginal dryness also occurs as estrogen levels drop off at menopause, a double whammy for women with diabetes. Some medications, such as those that cause dry mouth—antihistamines, some antidepressants, and some antihypertensives (medication to treat high blood pressure)—also can affect vaginal lubrication. Check with your doctor if you think your medication may be causing vaginal dryness. Many couples incorporate the use of water-based lubricants like K-Y jelly into their lovemaking. These products are safe to use and wash off easily.

Some women with diabetes also experience a decreased sex drive. The cause of diminished libido is difficult to pinpoint. Having a chronic disease like diabetes can cause anxiety, feelings of being less attractive, or even depression, all of which can affect desire. Sexual pleasure in part depends on feeling good about yourself and letting yourself go. Diabetes, by contrast, is all about control.

Sex, like other physical activity, can precipitate hypoglycemia. You may need to check your blood glucose level before and after intercourse, and have a snack, if necessary. Many women find that planning alleviates the fear of a hypoglycemic episode, which can affect sexual desire. If you use an insulin pump, you can disconnect it during sex, but remember to reconnect it within one hour.

These actions may seem to take away from spontaneity, but again, it's a matter of attitude. Diabetes is part of who you are, but in no way does it detract from the beautiful, loving person you are. Making love is about giving and receiving pleasure. Physical limitations may affect the ways you and your partner show affection, but they need not keep you from being sexually intimate.

Sexual fulfillment is an important part of being human. If you are having problems with sexual desire, arousal, or orgasms, talk to one of your health care providers. Many people are uncomfortable discussing sex with their doctors, but remember that your medical team is trained to discuss all aspects of your health and well-being. Sex is one pleasure that you do not have to sacrifice for diabetes.

6

Psychosocial Impact

Joyce is a customer service representative whose work is very stressful. Although she knows that as a woman with diabetes she has to lose weight, she finds comfort in food. She craves cookies and chips and often finds herself raiding the pantry when she comes home at night. She has learned, however, that she cannot keep junk food in the house and has stocked up on popcorn and other healthful snacks in an effort to manage her emotional eating.

Diabetes does not take a vacation. It is with you every hour of the day and every day of the week. It can be a frustrating disease. Sometimes, despite doing everything right, your blood glucose levels may still be high or you may develop complications. Other times, you may over-shoot your goal and have an episode of hypoglycemia. Diabetes can be overwhelming. Your doctor can't just control the disease for you; you must be responsible for managing the day-to-day aspects of your own care.

Chronic diseases like diabetes last a lifetime and can be controlled but not cured. Those facts alone can raise feelings of hopelessness, anger, and fear. Even in the best of times, life is filled with uncertainty and stress. Having diabetes makes it that much harder. On top of juggling other life responsibilities, you must now think about everything you eat, every activity you do or don't do, your schedule, and their combined effects on your blood sugar levels. You're expected to do a lot today and every day to ward off the future threat of complications.

Emotional, psychological, and social factors may affect your diabetes. Stress and overeating can raise your blood glucose levels. In addition, depression or anxiety can decrease your ability to take care of yourself properly. An estimated 10–30 percent of patients with diabetes experience depression. Depression is associated with higher-than-normal blood sugars for patients with type 1 or type 2 diabetes. Social factors—the support you do or do not get from your family; traditional ethnic diets; and society's expectation that a woman juggle multiple roles, for example—also affect your ability to manage your disease effectively.

In this chapter we discuss some of the psychosocial factors that accompany diabetes. Our hope is that this information will help you develop skills to cope with the daily burden of diabetes care, understand when to turn to friends, family, and professionals for help, and muster the inner strength to ensure that you, and not your diabetes, control your life.

ADJUSTMENT AFTER DIAGNOSIS

In Chapter 2 we touched on the roller coaster of feelings that can accompany a diagnosis of diabetes: shock, anger, fear, sadness or depression, and finally acceptance. You may have had no symptoms when you found out you had diabetes, and so the diagnosis didn't seem real. Then you were quickly confronted with massive amounts of information you needed to take care of yourself properly. Mastering it seemed overwhelming. Learning about the potential complications of the disease was probably very frightening.

The first year after diagnosis will require not only lifestyle adjustments but emotional adjustments as well. What you are feeling in part depends on what stage of life you're in at the time of diagnosis. If you're young and single, you might worry about attracting a mate and some day having children. It may feel like all your hopes and dreams are now unattainable. If you're at midlife, diabetes is another reminder that we don't live forever. You might worry about keeping your job and health insurance, and taking care of your family. If you have always been the pillar of strength in your family, you may fear that your illness will change family dynamics. If you develop diabetes during the later years of life, you may be faced with changing highly ingrained lifestyle behaviors. You may have been diagnosed after other losses in your life. Or you may know someone who lost her sight or a foot to diabetes and worry about that happening to you. Contemplating the new realities of your life can be distressing.

The diagnosis of diabetes brings the expectation that your lifestyle will have to change. While it is true that certain old behaviors will need to change and new daily chores will be added, your life is not over just because you now have diabetes. You will receive instructions from the diabetes nurse educator, your physician, and perhaps a dietitian on how to accomplish the necessary changes. In many areas of the country, programs are available to help you learn to manage the disease, which we'll talk about more in the next chapter.

Your life is not over just because you have diabetes.

But it's equally important to get assistance on coping emotionally with diabetes. If you're having trouble adjusting, you might be more susceptible to depression and anxiety down the road. Fluctuations in blood sugar levels alone can make you irritable, anxious, and depressed. Or you may have an underlying mood disorder, which can be triggered by the stresses of dealing with your diabetes diagnosis.

Coping difficulties can range from trouble dealing with daily hassles, constant worrying, sadness, and under- or overeating, to more paralyzing anxiety disorders, eating disorders, and major depression. Help is available for all these problems.

Ideally, a psychologist or social worker will be available as part of your diabetes care team. But if not, you should talk to a member of your health care team if your feelings affect your ability to function day to day. This is especially critical if your feelings are so intense that you want to skip your medication or harm yourself.

Support groups, and a new concept called group diabetes medical visits, are also helpful resources as you struggle to come to terms with your diagnosis. Diabetes group visits bring together people with chronic diseases who, led by a professional (usually a physician together with a nurse or psychologist), share their experiences and difficulties and work together to find healthier and more effective ways to cope. The diabetes group medical visit complements the individual medical visit and includes a brief medical evaluation to update medications, screening measures, diabetes goals, and treatment plans. Many people find emotional support just by being part of a group of people who uniquely understand what they're going through. Information and support are also available on the Internet, through professionally moderated discussion groups or bulletin boards.

DAILY HASSLES

Living with diabetes is like being sick but not sick. Unless your glucose control is poor or you are experiencing any medical complications, you feel pretty good most of the time. It's a disease that is largely invisible to others. But you know you have it and, as many women report, you "just don't feel right."

People will not always be understanding about what you can and can't do once you're diagnosed with diabetes. Sometimes you will have to deal with a lack of support from loved ones; at other times, your family may be too intrusive, for example, monitoring every morsel of food you eat or nagging you to exercise.

Whether they have type 1 or type 2 diabetes, most people find the day-to-day management of the disease challenging. There's a lot to remember to do, monitoring is time-consuming, and it can be unpleasant. It's easy to feel sorry for yourself. You might feel deprived because you shouldn't eat what you want to eat or, if you do, you feel guilty. If you must inject insulin, life gets even more complicated. The newer blood glucose monitoring machines are smaller than the older models and more convenient when you're on the go, but you must still prick your finger or another part of your body for blood. Despite all your best efforts, your blood glucose level may periodically be too high, too low, or erratic.

It is common to feel angry or frustrated, or to go through periods when you feel unmotivated to take care of yourself properly. We all "cheat" once in a while, but cheating can have serious consequences if you have diabetes. Many people are in denial when they are diagnosed and first experience a complication of the disease. You may hope your diabetes goes away (which of course it won't) and so pretend that nothing is wrong. Or you may convince yourself that you don't have time to deal with the disease now, and that you'll go to the doctor next month. Denial can be dangerous if it keeps you from getting the care you need.

Though you may not rid your life of anger, you can turn it to your advantage. Use it, for example, to drive your determination to reach your treatment goals.

Anger is also common. It seems grossly unfair to have diabetes. It changes your life. You can be so angry about the disease that you refuse to deal with it. But if you don't control your diabetes now, you will feel worse and increase your risk for problems down the road. Though you may not rid your life of anger, you can turn it to your advantage. Use it, for example, to drive your determination to reach your treatment goals.

Diabetes "burn-out" is another emotional pitfall of the relentless, demanding nature of this disease. You know what you need to do to control the disease, but you are just plain tired of doing it. You start checking your blood glucose levels less frequently—or not at all. Or, faced with some new expectation at work, in your family responsibilities, or in the self-management of your health care, you just throw up your hands in resignation.

Everyone's life is different, so the key to preventing burn-out or getting back on track will necessarily be different. But even if you are feeling overwhelmed by everything in your life, try to single out one specific problem or frustration. Then come up with a solution to that problem. Even one solution may be enough to get you back on an even keel again. If you're frustrated about high blood glucose levels, for example, ask your health care team for new strategies. If you're anxious about taking on an additional responsibility at home or work, talk to family or friends about helping with daily chores, or speak to your boss about adjusting your workload. If you're not getting any exercise, enlist a friend to walk regularly with you—someone to whom you can vent your feelings and share a laugh.

As bad as your frustration, anger, denial, and burn-out may be, they are even worse if you feel isolated, ashamed, or think you are the only one who experiences them. These feelings, in fact, are very common in men *and* women with diabetes.

Take a minute to do the self-assessment below to understand better how you are feeling. If you answer "yes" to any of the following questions, let your health care provider know at your next appointment:

➡ Do you find caring for your diabetes difficult because you do not feel any symptoms?
➡ Do you feel angry that you have diabetes?
➡ Are you scared because you have seen bad things happen to other people with diabetes?
➡ Are you in shock over the diagnosis?

➡ Are you afraid you will be a burden to your family?

➡ Does your family complain about what you have to do to manage your diabetes?

➡ Do you have a hard time contacting your medical providers?

THE STRESS EFFECT

Stress is an unfortunate by-product of our fast-paced, modern lifestyle. Studies have shown that people with diabetes who experience high levels of stress are at an increased risk for depression. You may experience stress if you're sick or injured. You will undoubtedly feel stressed if you are going through a divorce, dealing with a teenage child, acting as a single parent or a stepmother, having financial difficulties, feeling overworked, and so on. Living with a chronic disease with the specter of future medical problems can also be a major source of stress. Stress affects not only your ability to cope emotionally with diabetes and take care of yourself properly; it can also affect blood glucose levels.

Stress triggers a physiological response in the body, releasing hormones that ready us to deal with whatever made us scared or excited. Adrenaline, for example, causes the heart to beat faster, pumping blood more quickly through the body to the limbs. Glucose is released from storage sites for quick energy. Other hormones increase blood pressure and recruit white blood cells, which are involved in fighting infection.

Someone with diabetes may not have enough insulin available to deal with the extra glucose that is released, and so blood glucose levels may rise. Moreover, in those with type 2 diabetes, stress may interfere with the release of insulin. Research on the effects of stress on blood glucose has shown mixed results: the glucose levels of those with type 2 most often rise, but in people with type 1 glucose levels can go up or down. Either way, stress can upset the balance of diet, activity, and medications that keep both type 1 and type 2 diabetes under control.

SYMPTOMS OF STRESS

Anxiety

Twitching or trembling

Muscle tension, headaches

Sweating

Dry mouth, difficulty swallowing

Abdominal pain (especially in children)

Dizziness

Rapid or irregular heart rate

Rapid breathing

Diarrhea or frequent need to urinate

Fatigue

Irritability, including loss of temper

Sleeping difficulties and nightmares

Decreased concentration

Sexual problems

Source: Adapted from "Stress and Anxiety," MedlinePlus (www.nlm.nih.gov/medlineplus/ency/article/003211.htm).

Relaxation therapy and stress-management programs may help combat stress. These programs often include what's called "progressive muscle relaxation," in which you learn to relax muscles by tensing and releasing them one at a time, "mental imagery" (visualizing calming and peaceful places and things), and deep-breathing exercises.

Sometimes all it takes to manage stress is to find an activity, a hobby, or an exercise routine that relaxes you. Some forms of exercise, such as yoga and tai chi, combine movement with proper breathing, and emphasize keeping your mind centered on what you're doing rather than on your worries. Some women find it relaxing to listen to music, go out dancing, or shop. A massage can relieve stress.

Making time for yourself is not a luxury; it's a medical necessity.

WAYS TO REDUCE STRESS

Change your environment
Reduce external factors such as noise and pollution
Simplify your life at home when possible
Simplify your life at work when possible
Reduce threats to your physical safety
Change your behavior
Eat a balanced diet
Get enough sleep
Get adequate exercise
Learn relaxation techniques or meditation
Cut back on alcohol and caffeine consumption
Reduce exposure to situations that involve conflict
Take a time-management course
Undergo hypnosis
Develop a new attitude
Set limits for yourself and others
Become more aware of other options
Become more aware of what you are feeling
Be more willing to express your feelings
Become more confident about your own perceptions
Become more aware of the possibility of internal change

Source: K. J. Carlson, S. A. Eisenstat, and T. Ziporyn, *The New Harvard Guide to Women's Health* (Cambridge, Mass.: Harvard University Press, 2004), p. 575.

Plan an activity that makes you feel good. Even a half hour in a quiet room can be the reset button you need to face the world and its stressors again.

A positive attitude can also help reduce stress. If the source of your anxiety is traffic on the commute to work, maybe you can talk to your boss about driving in to work earlier and leaving earlier, or even working from home some of the time. Or perhaps you can decide that you're just not going to let the traffic bother you anymore. Turn on the radio and use the time to relax or plan. Change what you can change, and accept what you can't.

WHEN WORRY TAKES OVER

It is normal to feel anxious or nervous about financial difficulties or an important decision. Certainly the diagnosis of diabetes creates an overflow of worries as you adjust to your new realities. But some people experience an exaggerated response to worries or fears, which causes such distress that they cannot function properly. Worry can be beneficial if it prompts us to take action, to make healthier food choices, for example. But sometimes you can get locked into a cycle of futile worrying. You think about something over and over again without arriving at any solutions. You know you are needlessly tormenting yourself, but you can't stop. You may even be physically tense: you can't sleep; you get headaches, stomachaches, or tense muscles. You can't concentrate on other things.

If this describes you, then you may have an anxiety disorder. Women are slightly more prone to anxiety disorders than men, and the condition is even more prevalent among those with diabetes.

There are several kinds of anxiety disorders: generalized anxiety disorder, obsessive-compulsive disorder, panic disorder, social anxiety disorder, and post-traumatic stress disorder. Each has its own constellation of symptoms, but general symptoms include:

- ➡ feelings of panic, fear, and uneasiness
- ➡ obsessive thoughts and/or ritualistic behaviors, such as repeated hand washing
- ➡ problems sleeping, nightmares
- ➡ cold or sweaty hands
- ➡ shortness of breath, heart palpitations
- ➡ inability to be still and calm

➡ dry mouth
➡ muscle tension
➡ repeated thoughts or flashbacks of traumatic experiences

A hallmark of panic disorders, for example, is panic attacks, a sudden, intense feeling of anxiety along with at least four other symptoms: heart palpitations, chest tightness, dizziness, nausea, and fear of dying or losing control. Panic attacks are much more intense than feeling "stressed out" and can be confused with heart attacks. People who have occasional panic attacks may experience them in response to a particular stressor or a fearful situation. But someone with panic disorder has attacks that come unexpectedly in seemingly harmless situations. They may wake up in the middle of the night in sheer terror, only to have symptoms pass about ten minutes later. Or they might suddenly have a panic attack for no obvious reason when driving to work.

Someone with a social anxiety disorder fears embarrassment, humiliation, criticism, or drawing attention to his- or herself in social situations. This is different from having a social phobia, such as a fear of public speaking. It is also different from being shy or self-conscious about how you look. Someone with social anxiety disorder has an excessive fear and avoidance of meeting new people, parties, group meetings, any kind of confrontation, interactions with authority figures, or eating or drinking in public. Physical signs of such anxiety are blushing, sweating, trembling, and heart palpitations. Social anxiety disorder can significantly interfere with one's family and social life and with job advancement.

Anxiety disorders can be associated with depression or with alcohol abuse (drinking excessively to feel more comfortable socially, for example). Some women with anxiety disorders report that their symptoms worsen before their menstrual periods; it is even possible that you think you have PMS (premenstrual syndrome) when you really have an anxiety disorder or depression.

You can learn techniques to help you relax or to shift attention away from your worries. But true anxiety disorders cannot be wished away. They can be effectively treated, however, through psychotherapy and, depending on the severity of the anxiety, medication. (See Table 6.1 for a description of common medications used to treat depression and anxiety.)

WHEN FEELING DOWN IS DEPRESSION

Depression is even more common than anxiety disorders. It is the second most common diagnosis (after hypertension) made by primary care physicians, and women are at higher risk than men. In addition, if you have diabetes, you are twice as likely to suffer from depression as someone who does not have the disease.

It is important to know the symptoms of depression because, if left untreated, it can affect your ability to care for your diabetes. You may have several symptoms of depression—like an estimated 31 percent of all people with diabetes—or full-blown major depression, as 11 percent do. In either case, help is available. Treatment not only improves mood, but also seems to improve blood glucose control.

When we talk about depression, we don't mean having a bad day, feeling down, or grieving over a loss, which all of us experience at one time or another. Major depression is more chronic, recurrent, and intense, and is defined by having at least five of the symptoms listed below. For a clinician to consider a diagnosis of depression, one or both of the first two symptoms must be present for at least two weeks. Four other symptoms must be present as well:

- ➡ prolonged feelings of extreme sadness or hopelessness (every day, most of the day);
- ➡ significantly decreased interest or pleasure in activities that were once enjoyed;
- ➡ difficulty sleeping or sleeping more than usual nearly every day;
- ➡ fatigue or lack of energy;
- ➡ difficulty concentrating, remembering, or making decisions;

➡ significant weight loss, when not trying;

➡ restlessness, anxiety, irritability;

➡ recurring thoughts of death or suicide;

➡ constant feelings of worthlessness or inappropriate guilt.

Some of the symptoms—such as fatigue and weight loss—can be associated with high glucose levels and don't necessarily mean you are depressed, unless you have other symptoms as well.

Major depression is the most serious depressive disorder but not the only one. Dysthymic disorder is diagnosed when someone has experienced a depressed mood more days than not for at least two years, in addition to at least two of the symptoms listed above (one of the two could also be low self-esteem). "Adjustment disorder with a depressed mood" is considered when someone has more difficulty than should be expected coping with a stressful event, such as the diagnosis of diabetes, divorce, or the death of a loved one.

If you are experiencing any of these symptoms, talk with someone on your health care team. He or she can evaluate you for depression or refer you to someone who can. Because depression affects a person's ability to function in everyday life, someone who is depressed is probably not controlling her diabetes as well as she could. This situation not only increases the risk of complications but also adds further stress and can worsen the depression.

Psychotherapy, antidepressants, support groups, or a combination of these approaches can successfully treat most cases of depression. The newest antidepressants, the selective serotonin reuptake inhibitors (SSRIs), are as effective as older antidepressants but are less likely to cause weight gain or drowsiness or affect your blood sugar. They do have other side effects, however, as shown in Table 6.1.

We don't know why women, and those with diabetes in particular, are more prone to depression than men. Although coping with diabetes and its complications contributes to depression, it cannot fully explain the connection. In fact, in the vast majority of people with type 2 diabetes who also have depression, the depression came before

Table 6.1 Antidepression and antianxiety medications

Drug	Dose range (mg/day)	Side effects (apply to all drugs in class)	Recommended use (apply to all drugs in class)
Serotonin reuptake inhibitors (SSRI)			
Citalopram (Celexa)	20–60	sedation, decreased	depression, panic
Fluoxetine (Prozac)	10–80	libido	disorder, social anxiety,
Fluvoxamine (Luvox)	50–300		general anxiety,
Paroxetine (Paxil)	10–50		premenstrual syndrome,
Sertraline (Zoloft)	25–200		some chronic pain syndromes like neuropathy
Escitalopram (Lexapro)	10–20	sometimes nausea	depression
Tricyclic antidepressants (TCA)*			
Amitriptyline (Elavil)	50–300	weight gain, sedation,	depression, general
Clomipramine (Anafranil)	25–250	hyperglycemia	anxiety, some chronic
Desipramine (Norpramin)	150–300		pain syndromes
Monoamine oxidase inhibitor (MAOIs)*			
Phenelzine (Nardil)	45–90	multiple drug and diet interactions	panic disorder, social anxiety, general anxiety
Buspirone (BuSpar)	15–60		panic disorder, social anxiety, general anxiety
Beta blockers			
Propanolol (Inderal)	10–160	depression, sedation	social anxiety, high blood pressure, prevention of headaches
Benzodiazepines (BZD)			
Alprazolam (Xanax)	2–10	memory problems,	panic disorder, general
Clonazepam (Klonopin)	1–5	abuse potential, need	anxiety, social anxiety
Lorazepam (Ativan)	3–12	to wean off	

Drug	Dose range (mg/day)	Side effects	Recommended use
Mirtazapine (Remeron)	15–45	sedation	depression
Nefazodone (Serzone)	300–600	sedation	depression
Venlafaxine (Effexor XR)	75–375	jitteriness, upset stomach, high blood pressure	panic disorder, general anxiety, postmenopausal hot flashes
Bupropion (Wellbutrin, Wellbutrin SR, Wellbutrin XL, Zyban)	150–450	dry mouth, nausea, seizures (rare)	depression, general anxiety, smoking cessation

* These medications must be used with caution in people with diabetes. For additional information about medications, see www.nlm.nih.gov/medlineplus.

the diagnosis of diabetes. Depression may in some way increase insulin resistance (the same may be true for bipolar disorder, commonly known as manic depression). Or someone with type 1 or type 2 diabetes may have a genetic predisposition to depression. We know that some women are especially sensitive to the hormonal changes that occur in the menstrual cycle, and are more prone to PMS, postpartum depression (depression that occurs after having a baby), and depression during perimenopause.

Studies have found associations between depression and obesity, physical inactivity, cigarette smoking, and substance abuse. Depression is also linked to an increased risk of cardiovascular disease.

Even women whose symptoms aren't severe enough to qualify for the diagnosis of depression may benefit from counseling. How well you feel emotionally influences how well you feel physically—and vice versa.

THE EXTRA WEIGHT OF OBESITY

Ironically, though our society idealizes thinness, two-thirds of all Americans are overweight or obese. Many, particularly women, are not happy about it, and dieting has become a national obsession. Broadly speaking, just being obese does not make someone more susceptible to depression and other mental illnesses. But certain subgroups of obese people are at increased risk for depression: women, people who "binge eat," and those who are extremely obese.

Obese women are more likely than average-weight women or obese men to be depressed and more likely to have an eating disorder called "binge eating" (described in the next section). Women are more apt than men to be teased or ridiculed about their weight and to report less satisfaction with their bodies. A negative body image has been linked to depression and low self-esteem.

More than 90 percent of people with type 2 diabetes are at least overweight (defined as a BMI of 25 or more) and nearly half are obese.

Obesity is defined as a body mass index that is greater than or equal to 30 kg/m (a woman who is 5'6" with a BMI of 30, for example, would weigh 186 pounds). (See Appendix 1.)

Losing weight requires significant behavioral changes. Adjusting your lifestyle can be extremely stressful, especially for women who may have already tried and failed to lose weight many times. Repeated cycles of weight loss and regain are associated with decreased satisfaction with appearance, self-esteem, and self-confidence.

To succeed at weight loss, you will need to treat any existing depression, anxiety, or eating disorders. Reducing psychological distress sets a better stage for accomplishing your goals. You'll need a great deal of motivation and self-confidence to change ingrained eating behaviors. But success has both physical and emotional rewards.

ALCOHOL AND DRUG USE

Drug and alcohol abuse is not more prevalent among people with diabetes. But because dependence on these substances can have debilitating effects on diabetes care and health in general, it is important to discuss them.

As long as you account for the calories or carbohydrates in your meal plan, a moderate amount of alcohol in your diet is fine. Though not a reason to start drinking, research shows that drinking moderate amounts of alcohol, particularly red wine, can actually lower your risk of heart disease. Moderate usually means one drink a day for women: 5 ounces of wine, 12 ounces of beer (one bottle), or a mixed drink containing 1.5 ounces of "hard liquor," such as scotch, vodka, or gin. Remember that each of these drinks has about 100 to 150 calories, and mixers can add even more calories (see Table 6.2). Drinking alcohol can be counterproductive if you are trying to decrease calories to lose weight.

Alcohol may precipitate or worsen a hypoglycemic episode if you take insulin or a sulfonylurea. If you take one of these medicines, it

Table 6.2   Calories in alcoholic beverages

Beverage	Calories per 1 fluid oz.	Average serving size	Total calories
Beer (regular)	12	12 oz.	144
Beer (light)	9	12 oz.	108
White wine	20	5 oz.	105
Red wine	21	5 oz.	105
Sweet dessert wine	47	3 oz.	141
80 proof distilled spirits (gin, rum, vodka, whiskey)	64	1.5 oz.	96

Source: "Dietary Guidelines for Americans," USDA (www.health.gov/dietaryguidelines/dga2005/document/html/chapter9.htm).

is a good idea to eat food when you drink. You should mention to your physician how much you typically drink, as alcohol may affect your blood sugar control. Chronic, heavy drinking may worsen specific complications of diabetes, such as neuropathy. Other health problems increase substantially above moderate levels of drinking.

Women represent about one-third of those with alcohol abuse or dependence problems in the United States. Women metabolize alcohol differently from men, in part because of their smaller size, with the result that drinking may have a greater effect on a woman's body. Women are also more apt to use alcohol to reduce stress. There is a link between eating disorders (particularly bulimia) and alcohol and drug problems in women. Depression and anxiety disorders can also occur in conjunction with alcohol abuse.

Often what begins as occasional use of a recreational drug to feel good becomes an all-consuming addiction, resulting in legal and interpersonal problems, unfulfilled work and family responsibilities, and, in the case of diabetes, poor management of the disease. Prescription drugs can be abused if not used as originally intended. Pain medications and some prescribed antianxiety medications and diet medications can be addictive as well. Then there are the illegal street drugs that we typically associate with abuse and addiction: marijuana, cocaine, heroin, and ecstasy.

It is very hard for someone to recognize when her own use of al-

SIGNS OF ALCOHOL ABUSE

Primary care physicians use the following questions, known as the CAGE questionnaire, to determine if a woman might have an alcohol problem:

Cut Down: Have you ever tried to cut down on your drinking?

Annoyed: Have you ever been annoyed by criticism of your drinking?

Guilt: Have you ever felt guilty about your drinking?

Eye opener: Have you ever had an eye opener (a drink first thing in the morning)?

If you answered yes to any of these questions, talk to your health care team.

cohol or another drug has become abuse. If a friend or family member has expressed concern, if you find your day revolving around a drug or drink, if you find yourself lying or making excuses or hiding your use, take a hard look at yourself. It is time to talk to someone on your health care team about the possibility of a problem.

A DANGEROUS DUO: DIABETES AND EATING DISORDERS

Women of all ethnic and racial groups are prone to unhealthful eating patterns. Even in some African American and Latin cultures, where a larger body size is traditionally more accepted than waif-like thinness, women are getting swept up in mainstream society's preoccupation with slimness. Consequently, it is no longer just the stereotypical young, white female seeking perfection who has an eating disorder.

Eating disorders and diabetes are a dangerous duo. Body-image problems are a central feature of eating disorders, and having diabetes can heighten the feeling that one's body is defective. An alarmingly high number of teenage girls and young adult women with type 1 diabetes are "insulin purging," skipping or reducing their insulin doses to lose weight. Binge eating is also common among women with type 1 diabetes, and it is the main eating disorder afflicting women with type 2. These practices can wreak havoc on blood glucose levels and long-term health.

A case could be made that very little healthful eating goes on in this country. Overeating is rampant. Most women are preoccupied with food and weight and many occasionally binge or purge themselves. But eating disorders represent the dangerous extremes of unhealthful eating. There are three types of eating disorders:

ANOREXIA NERVOSA. In pursuit of thinness, women with anorexia severely restrict their food intake, often consuming as few as two hundred calories a day, and may exercise compulsively. Their body image is so distorted that they think they are fat even when they are so emaciated that their health is in danger. Anorexia nervosa is relatively rare but can be life-threatening.

BULIMIA NERVOSA. After uncontrolled binging on large quantites of food, women with bulimia "purge" by vomiting, taking laxatives or diuretics, exercising excessively, or, in the case of diabetics, not taking insulin.

BINGE EATING DISORDER. Women (and men) with binge eating disorder binge uncontrollably at one sitting, at least twice a week, and are distressed about it, but they don't try to rid their body of the food just eaten. Binge eating is common.

We should note that the majority of overweight or obese people do not regularly binge on huge quantities of food. Most eat slightly more calories than they expend on a daily basis; over years, their body weight slowly increases. But among those who seek professional weight-loss treatment, anywhere from 7 percent to 19 percent are found to binge eat. Studies have shown that between 6 and 25 percent of people with type 2 diabetes suffer from binge eating disorder. The prevalence of the disorder appears to increase in the higher weight ranges. Binge eating is also extremely common among girls and women with type 1 diabetes. Some use fear of hypoglycemia, low blood glucose, as an excuse to overeat.

Binge eaters are more likely than others to have low self-esteem, body-image dissatisfaction, and symptoms of depression or other mental illnesses. Binge eating raises blood glucose levels and causes weight gain, which in turn increases insulin resistance and worsens diabetes.

Research has shown that once a binge-eating cycle is stopped and a more regular pattern of eating is started, women feel less hungry, less deprived, and have fewer negative feelings about food and eating. In turn, reducing hunger and negative feelings, which are thought to lead to binge eating in the first place, decreases the frequency of binges.

About one-third of all women with type 1 diabetes will occasionally omit insulin intentionally. Sometimes insulin is omitted because of the fear of hypoglycemia, but in young women, weight loss is often the motivation. Adolescent girls and young adult women with diabetes have received the greatest attention because they appear to be the most susceptible to full-blown eating disorders, perhaps twice as likely as women their age without diabetes. But even disordered eating that is not consistent or severe enough to earn a diagnostic label of an eating disorder can be harmful to current and future health.

Maintaining blood glucose levels close to normal clearly prevents or slows the progression of diabetes-related complications. Unfortunately, improving blood glucose control often causes an initial weight gain. If someone with diabetes doesn't have enough insulin to escort glucose into the cells of the body that need it, the glucose levels rise in the blood and glucose is urinated out. Calories, in the form of glucose, are lost. In addition, water is lost. The end result is that poorly controlled diabetes is associated with weight loss.

When control of glucose levels improves, you may gain weight because now your body is able to use the glucose rather than expelling it in the urine. You are now also retaining the fluids you need to stay hydrated.

Careful meal planning and exercise can limit weight gain. But some girls and women get into a pattern of omitting or reducing the amount of insulin they need in order to lose weight. This "insulin purging" puts them at risk for ketoacidosis (an emergency situation when blood sugars and breakdown products from fat get too high; see Chapter 4) and, in the long run, for diabetic complications. Cutting down on insulin doses is a dangerous practice, and once it becomes a habit, it is very difficult to stop without professional help.

Women engaged in disordered eating practices are often ashamed and embarrassed to mention the problem to their health care practitioners. Just remember that food issues are very common among women in our society. Sharing the problem with a professional who can help you address it can be a big relief.

SIGNS OF A PROBLEM

Food can become all-consuming, all you think about. Below is a quiz prepared by the Joslin Diabetes Center that may help you determine if you have eating issues that you should discuss with a member of your health care team:

➡ Do you frequently lose weight only to regain it?
➡ Have you been on five or more weight-loss diets in the past five years?
➡ Do you think you have a problem with food?
➡ Do you eat large amounts of food in a short space of time?
➡ Do you have trouble controlling the amount you eat?
➡ Do you seem to constantly crave food?
➡ Do you eat until you feel uncomfortably full?
➡ Does your eating always seem to interfere with your diabetes control?
➡ Has your weight ever affected any part of your life?
➡ Do you weigh yourself every day? More than once a day?
➡ Do you often eat more than you planned to eat?

➡ Do you worry about your weight or body size?

➡ How many of these methods of weight loss have your tried?
- diuretics/laxatives
- self-induced vomiting
- fasting/starvation
- amphetamines or over-the-counter diet pills
- compulsive exercise
- insulin manipulation
- liquid diets (supervised or unsupervised)
- hypnosis
- special foods and drinks from individual weight-loss programs

➡ Do you prefer to eat alone?

➡ Do you avoid mirrors?

MOOD AND FOOD

Just try to find a woman in North America who has not eaten the equivalent of a pint of ice cream after the break-up of a relationship or some other emotional upset. Most women can identify with emotional eating, using food to provide comfort, ease stress, or relieve boredom. This is eating not out of hunger but in response to emotions such as sadness, loneliness, anxiety, stress, or frustration. As the joke goes, "stressed" spelled backwards is "desserts."

Having diabetes doesn't make you any different from any other woman on that account. But diabetes does make it all the more important for you to sort out what provokes emotional eating and to try to omit it. Emotional eating may be a big reason for your weight gain over the years, which in turn has led to high glucose levels, and perhaps high blood pressure and cholesterol as well. Emotional eating becomes a habit, which must be recognized before it can be broken.

One of the reasons that women enrolled in the Diabetes Prevention Program successfully lost weight was that they received intensive counseling about eating behaviors. They learned how to identify pat-

---

WEIGHT-LOSS TIPS

• Post a sign on your refrigerator door: Am I Really Hungry?
• Try to avoid television or other activities that cause you to eat more.
• Don't keep junk food in the house.

---

terns of behavior that led to weight gain, how to problem-solve, and how to establish new habits and more positive ways of thinking about food.

Here's an example used in the DPP's lifestyle-intervention training sessions:

Sarah is a busy woman with a job and a family. Yesterday she was extremely busy at work and didn't eat lunch because she didn't have time to go out. In the afternoon, her boss was very critical and demanding, and Sarah felt stressed and anxious. At the end of the day, Sarah came home tired, upset, and hungry. She went right to the kitchen. She immediately saw a package of cookies on the kitchen counter, and before she knew it, she had eaten a fair number of the cookies.

This example was used in a behavioral support session to illustrate problem-solving as a way to stop unhealthful eating. Participants would have been asked to identify the problem in this example, what led up to it, and ways to change the end result at various links in the chain of events.

Using the DPP example, let's identify some things in Sarah's day that led up to her emotional eating. Each provides an opportunity to change the final outcome next time around. She didn't eat lunch, for example. We know that spreading the food you eat throughout the day and not skipping meals is key to not overeating later (as is eating smaller portions more slowly). Skipping meals regularly causes the body to slow its metabolism to conserve, rather than burn, calories. Also, Sarah bought cookies and left them out. Another solution would be to buy low-calorie snacks like fruit and eat them next time she comes home upset.

This example could also be used to think about alternative ways to relieve stress. Perhaps Sarah needs to talk with her boss and clearly communicate to him that his expectations are unfair. Or perhaps, if she had just taken the lunch break she was due, she would have been better able to deal with her boss's demands later in the day. When she got home, she could have tried nonfood ways to relieve her stress: a hot shower, calling a friend to vent, writing in a journal, pulling weeds, or even screaming into a pillow.

Ask yourself, do I eat more when I am stressed out? Do I change the kinds of foods I eat? What could I do instead to relieve stress the next time I feel the urge to reach for the cookies?

When we eat out of boredom, sadness, or stress we tend to get down on ourselves. We think, "I'll never be able to lose weight. I don't have will power. I'm a failure. I might as well eat some more." Then an episode of overeating becomes an excuse to slip off a meal plan. This habit can be broken. Participants in the Diabetes Prevention Program learned how to "talk back" to their negative thoughts. They were told to picture a giant, red stop sign to stop the negative thought. Then they replaced it with a positive thought: It takes time to make lifelong changes. Slips are normal and to be expected. My next meal will be a healthy one.

These examples illustrate how behavioral support might help you overcome personal hurdles to losing weight. If weight loss is your goal, your diabetes nurse educator or dietitian can help you find a behavioral support program in your area.

From the body's standpoint, food may merely be fuel. But for many of us, eating and mealtimes play other roles. Dinners with family and friends are opportunities to reconnect after long, hectic days at work and school, or to catch up with people we don't see as often as we'd like. We want to be able to continue doing that without feeling deprived. A common reason for not sticking with a diet is the temptation that accompanies eating out at a restaurant or indulging at a party (we'll offer tips on how to handle such situations in Chapter 8). Another reason is social pressure from others. You can learn how to respond when someone repeatedly asks you, for example, if you want a piece of the pie she made. You can gently remind her that she is not being supportive. By serving healthful, tasty meals at your house, you can be a positive role model for family and friends—while still enjoying their company.

THE SUPERWOMAN COMPLEX

One of the most common problems facing women today is not a disorder you'll find in the medical textbooks. The Superwoman Complex is another product of our harried, modern society. Women—regardless of race, ethnicity, or social class—are juggling many roles. They are wives, mothers, employees and employers, and caregivers for aging parents. They are often exhausted and are used to putting everyone else's needs before their own.

But diabetes cannot take a backseat. You will not be able to take care of your numerous other responsibilities if you don't take care of yourself first. Think of the safety instructions given before every airplane takes off: if oxygen is required in the event of an emergency, put your mask on first, then help your children or others put theirs on. To help others, you must first be fully functioning yourself.

To provide adequate self-care you may need to ask for or accept help from family and friends. This is more difficult for some women than for others. Personal temperament, notions of a woman's role, and cultural expectations may make it hard for some women to reach out to others.

FAMILY, COMMUNITY, AND CULTURE

We have recently come to recognize that behaviors related to health and illness must be understood in the context of ethnicity, social class, gender, and family. These factors contribute to a woman's attitudes toward disease, the stressors in her life, her style of coping, and the amount and kind of support she receives from others.

Studies of African American women, for example, have pointed to racism and sexism as underlying stressors over which they feel little control. It has been suggested that some women cope by overperforming in their family role, and by trying to appear in control and poised at all times. There is a cultural expectation that an African American woman be a strong matriarch who sacrifices her needs for the family's. If this sounds like you, you could be giving yourself less-than-ideal care.

Your cultural heritage can influence how you respond to a crisis, such as a chronic illness like diabetes. Some Latinos, for example, believe that diabetes is their destiny, something they must simply accept. Others have the misconception that insulin causes blindness. Cultural heritage may partially explain why one person reacts stoically to pain and another reacts dramatically.

If you were born in another country and don't speak English very well, it is very important that you have a health care provider who speaks your language—or at least a translator who can. Educational materials about diabetes are now available in many languages, too.

Ideally, your health care providers should have some understanding of the different worldview that someone with a strong cultural identity brings with her diagnosis. If your ancestors were Northern Plains American Indians, for example, you might believe that all life is interrelated, and that people are to be seen not as individuals but as part of all creation. To be healthy requires harmony of the four components of one's being: mental, physical, emotional, and spiritual. You may perceive change as part of the circle of life. If so, you have a right to expect that someone helping you to cope emotionally with diabetes will respect these concepts.

As much as male/female role expectations have changed in the melting pot of modern American society, there is still a lingering, traditional expectation that women do most of the housekeeping, even if they also work outside the home. Clearly, with the addition of diabetes to the equation, you can't handle all your household duties and be expected to manage your diabetes without help. Your housework can wait a couple of days, but taking care of your diabetes cannot.

Family support in general is considered a critical factor in determining how well someone takes care of his or her diabetes. Women with diabetes may see offers of help as a challenge to their autonomy and independence. But people want to be of assistance. It's better to think of ways you would like them to help than to have them "help" in ways you don't welcome. For example, most people with diabetes resent efforts to police their food choices, no matter how well-meaning.

Here are some ways that friends or family members can support a woman with diabetes:

- Help plan meals, shop for groceries, or cook (keeping diabetes and obesity issues in mind).
- Learn how to respond to the most common emergencies: low or high blood sugars.
- Volunteer to walk or exercise regularly with her; you'll both benefit!
- Transport and accompany her to health care check-ups; listen, take notes, and ask questions.
- If she can't reach her feet to do a foot inspection, do it for her; massage her feet.
- Ask her how she's coping with her diabetes. Listen if she feels like talking about it, but don't press if she doesn't. Ask again another time.
- Offer to run errands for her, watch her children, or take a stint caring for the elderly parent in her care.

Diabetes is a difficult adjustment for everyone in the family. Loved ones might feel anger, frustration, and burn-out, too. After all, diabetes doesn't take a vacation for them, either.

FOCUS ON THE POSITIVE

Some days will be easier than others. You're on target for meeting your diabetes care goals, you're confident, and life is good. Other days you feel out of whack, you're irritable, you're not eating right, and life seems futile. Everyone has days like that. Remember that it could be the disease talking, telling you to bring your blood glucose down or up, for example. But it becomes a problem if a day or so of feeling bad stretches into weeks or months.

Sometimes the solution is as simple as putting your worries in perspective. Rather than feeling sorry for yourself, try focusing on what is positive in your life, or tapping your inner strength. More serious problems are not so easily solved, however, and require professional support and even medication.

Use the information in this chapter to hold a mirror up to yourself. Do you recognize yourself in any of the lists of warning signs? Is the way you're eating or the way you're feeling keeping you from meeting your goals? If the answer is yes, then maybe it's time to get some outside help. Mention your concerns to someone on your health care team. The mind is powerful and can work against you or for you.

7

Management of the Disease

Sylvia is relieved to hear that her HgbA$_{1c}$ is 6.5 percent. She has been working very hard to keep her sugars in good control. She joined a weight-loss program that provides her with meal plans, and she attends an aerobics class on the weekends at the local YMCA. She feels better eating healthful foods and has even grown to love fish, which she never thought would happen. She still has trouble remembering to check her glucose at bedtime, but she now sets her watch alarm in case she falls asleep after an exhausting day.

Your physician will not just hand you a prescription for medication to take three times a day—or at least he or she shouldn't. Diabetes care is unfortunately not that easy. But it doesn't have to disrupt your whole life, either. You can learn to integrate the demands of diabetes into your current lifestyle. Rather than the "do-as-I-say" approach, physicians now generally try to equip people with the know-how and tools to self-manage their disease in partnership with their medical team.

Self-management is based on the premise that on a daily basis *you* are the one in control of your diabetes. Since diabetes control is so integrally related to your lifestyle, it makes sense for you, not the doctors or nurses sitting in their offices, to make the onsite, minute-to-minute decisions. Your health care team educates, coaches, and actively communicates with you, but diabetes care is largely self-care.

With diabetes self-management education, you will learn what you have to do to control the disease, the pay-offs if you do, and the consequences if you don't. Your team may recommend a change in your current lifestyle—diet, activity levels, and schedule—but it will only happen when you yourself are committed to doing it.

What does self-management really mean? It empowers you to be an active partner with your health care providers in setting and reaching achievable goals based on the realities of your particular life. If you work, have children to care for, have food preferences and meal schedules, and have little time to exercise, for example, your health care providers will work with you to devise a diabetes care plan that accommodates these demands.

Your diabetes care plan is a work in progress. If you're not reaching your goal for glucose levels, it doesn't mean you're not working hard enough or have failed. It means the plan isn't working and needs to be tweaked. Here's an example of how a plan might be modified to better suit a busy lifestyle:

Donna has type 2 diabetes and works two jobs, as a secretary during the day and as a waitress on Friday and Saturday nights. She was finding it hard to meet her blood glucose goals because she was skipping meals during the day and snacking on weekends when she was at the restaurant. Her medical team worked with her to refine her meal plan. Since then, Donna has started to eat breakfast in the morning, bring a bag lunch to work, and carry a glucose monitor small enough to fit in her pocket. With more consistency in her meals, her blood sugar levels are better. She has even lost a few pounds with all the running around she's doing.

Overall, the goals of self-management are to feel well, avoid acute metabolic emergencies, and prevent or delay long-term complications. Whether you have type 1 or type 2 diabetes, managing your disease will require you to do the following:

→ Monitor blood glucose levels.
→ Achieve acceptable control of glucose levels through diet, activity, and by taking any prescribed medications such as oral medications and insulins.
→ Follow lifestyle recommendations and take prescribed medications to control other risk factors, such as high blood pressure and abnormal lipids, for long-term complications.
→ See your health care team regularly so they can screen for and manage complications.
→ Follow a recommended schedule of health care visits, tests, and immunizations.

In this chapter we present an overview of the nuts and bolts of care. This information is meant to complement, not replace, the advice and counsel of your medical team. Think of this as a roadmap of what you need to do to stay on the path to better diabetes control.

MONITORING BLOOD GLUCOSE LEVELS

In Chapter 4 we explained why glucose control is critical. In this chapter we describe how to achieve it. Glucose control hinges on striving for levels of glucose that are as close to the nondiabetic range as safely possible. A normal pancreas makes constant adjustments to the amount of insulin it produces to ensure that there's enough, but not too much, to do its job—escorting glucose and other nutrients out of the blood-stream and into the cells of the body, where they are needed for energy and growth. To accomplish this goal and imitate the nondiabetic pancreas, you first have to know how much glucose is in your blood at key times during the day.

In a person without diabetes, glucose is lower before meals and particularly after sleeping (a natural state of fasting) and higher right after meals. The glucose levels of someone with type 2 diabetes follow a similar pattern except that they tend to run 50 to even 200 or more points higher than in someone without diabetes. With type 2 diabetes, levels of glucose not only rise higher after meals but also remain higher for a longer period of time after the meal. The pancreas produces insulin, but not enough to overcome the insulin resistance.

By contrast, people with type 1 diabetes have much more erratic levels of glucose throughout the day because they are totally dependent on the doses of insulin they take, balanced with other factors like diet and activity that affect glucose levels. As a result, women with type 1 diabetes need to check how much glucose is in their blood at least four times a day, usually before meals and at bedtime, and sometimes two hours after eating. Frequent measurements are necessary to maintain intensive control and to adjust premeal insulin doses (see Table 7.1). In addition, if you have type 1 diabetes you will need to be sure your glucose level does not fall too low, especially after exercise or changes in your schedule. You may need to test more often if you are pregnant (see Chapter 5) or ill (Chapter 8).

Although most self-testing is to measure blood glucose levels, you may need to test your urine for ketones—breakdown products of fat that increase when diabetes is severely out of control—when you are ill or when your blood sugars are consistently higher than 300. If the urine strip shows more than a small amount of ketones, call your health care team immediately.

Table 7.1 Sample schedules for blood glucose self-monitoring

Type of treatment	Monitoring schedule
Diet alone	As needed
Oral medication	1–2 times a day[a,b]
Once-a-day insulin injection	1–2 times a day[a]
Twice-a-day insulin injections	2–4 times a day
Intensive insulin[c] or insulin pump	3–6 times a day

a. Can decrease to two to three times per week if stable.

b. May not need glucose monitoring if drugs that cause hypoglycemia (sulfonylureas or meglitinides) are not used.

c. Usually a long-acting basal insulin and a very rapid–acting insulin with meals (3–4 injections per day).

Source: Adapted from Silvio Inzucchi, *Diabetes Facts and Guidelines, 2002–2003*, Yale Diabetes Center.

With type 2 diabetes, glucose levels are more stable than with type 1, and so less frequent testing is required. If your diabetes is stable with diet alone or with a medication that doesn't cause hypoglycemia, you may need to monitor only when sick or if you develop symptoms that suggest high blood sugars. Your health care team will track your glucose control with other laboratory tests (see the discussion of HgbA$_{1c}$ that follows). Women with type 2 diabetes treated with insulin or a sulfonylurea medication (both of which can cause hypoglycemia) may need to measure glucose levels once or twice a day. You may have to test more often if you are pregnant, if you change medications or dosages, or if you have unusual stress or an illness. It is also a good idea to test your glucose before driving or performing any other potentially hazardous activity, to forestall an episode of hypoglycemia.

Self-monitoring of blood glucose is done with a portable glucose meter, which we'll describe a little later. The technology to self-monitor blood glucose has revolutionized the care of diabetes since its introduction in the late 1970s. It has largely replaced testing of urine for sugar levels, which was an indirect measure of blood glucose levels, could not tell you when blood glucose levels were less than 180 mg/dl, and, most notably, could not warn you of hypoglycemia.

The HgbA$_{1c}$, or glycohemoglobin, is a laboratory test that reflects average blood sugar levels over the previous two to three months. The test is usually performed every three or four months as part of a regular medical appointment and is used to determine if you are achieving the long-term sugar control required to prevent or delay the development of complications. The HgbA$_{1c}$ is also a useful way to double-check the accuracy of self-monitoring results, though it is no substitute for self-testing. Some home HgbA$_{1c}$ kits are now available, but most health care providers still do the test in a laboratory. Check with someone from your health care team before using one of these kits.

GLUCOSE GOALS

The major reason to do an HgbA$_{1c}$ test is to see if you are reaching the overall goals for diabetes control. People without diabetes will have an HgbA$_{1c}$ of 4 to 6 percent. The usual goal for those with diabetes is to achieve an HgbA$_{1c}$ as close to the nondiabetic range as safely possible, but no higher than 7 percent. The higher the HgbA$_{1c}$, the greater the risk of developing long-term complications.

In the nondiabetic person, blood glucose levels stay within narrow limits throughout the day. However, if you have diabetes, your blood sugar levels will be higher and fluctuate more, particularly if you have type 1. Even with good control of the disease, blood sugar levels will often drift outside the normal range. The aim is to keep your blood glucose on most days from rising too high, especially after meals, or too low.

The large clinical trials have shown us that the closer your HgbA$_{1c}$ is to 7 percent or less, the lower your risk for microvascular complications (retinopathy, neuropathy, and nephropathy) and, at least in type 1 diabetes, cardiovascular disease (heart attacks and stroke). In type 1 diabetes, for each 10 percent reduction in HgbA$_{1c}$—from 10 percent to 9 percent or from 9 to 8.1—there is a 43 percent reduction in diabetic eye disease. Similar beneficial effects of lowering blood glucose levels have been shown for type 2 diabetes.

To achieve a goal of 7 percent or less, you must strive for the following levels of plasma glucose when self-monitoring:

➡ 80–120 mg/dl before breakfast and other meals

➡ less than 180 mg/dl 90 to 120 minutes after meals, when your blood sugar usually peaks

Sometimes you will also need to test at bedtime, when your goal should be 90–180 mg/dl, depending on how close bedtime is to dinner. Bedtime blood glucose may be kept a little higher than daytime levels because of safety considerations. Testing may also be necessary if you are not feeling well or are concerned about your sugar level.

You'll be keeping a log book or diary of your blood glucose readings, so you and your health care team can check for patterns and determine if your treatment needs to be changed. In the log book you will record your glucose readings, what you ate that day, and any medications taken. It is also helpful to include comments about how you are feeling or about any symptoms you might be having. This information will help your medical provider analyze the data.

THE METER'S RUNNING

To self-monitor blood glucose you will need a glucose meter. There are more than twenty-five different glucose meters on the market to choose from (see Appendix 4 for a comparison chart). Most are portable and run on batteries. Current meters are small (about the size of a small cell phone), fast (requiring only five to fifteen seconds for a test), and accurate. At most, you will need only a very small drop of blood, obtained with a finger prick that is only minimally uncomfortable. Meters differ in cost, testing speed, whether or not they can store results, and the amount (and site) of the blood needed for an accurate reading.

We recommend that you consult your medical provider or diabetes nurse educator and take the time to find the meter that best suits your needs. You should consider ease of use, the visual display, memory functions, and portability. You should also check with your insurance company to determine which brands of meters are covered by

Blood sugar log

Date	Medication (dose)	Breakfast	Lunch	Dinner	Bedtime
Sunday	NPH 2X daily AM 22 PM 16	118	124	109	112
Comments: Felt really good today					
Monday	NPH 2X daily AM 22 PM 16	106	114	116	130
Comments:					
Tuesday	NPH 2X daily AM 22 PM 16	120	155*	139	128
Comments: *Glass of juice mid-morning					
Wednesday	NPH 2X daily AM 22 PM 16	111	140	120	116
Comments:					
Thursday	NPH 2X daily AM 22 PM 16	108	140	178*	137
Comments: *Ate out at office party					
Friday	NPH 2X daily AM 22 PM 16	103	117	142	129
Comments:					
Saturday	NPH 2X daily AM 22 PM 16	125	131	127	128
Comments: Felt good, took lunch time walk					

Keeping a log of your blood glucose readings will help you and your health care team determine if any treatment changes are necessary. Bring the log with you to every medical visit.

your plan. In some states, companies will come to your house and teach you how to use your glucose monitor.

Also note that the model of meter you choose will require its own brand of test strips. The cost of these test strips can vary, so do your research before deciding which model to go with. Most health in-

SELF-TESTING YOUR BLOOD GLUCOSE

If you're using your blood glucose meter for the first time, read the directions and store the meter where you can easily retrieve it.

1. If your hands are not clean, wash them with soap and warm water. You don't have to use an alcohol wipe.
2. Check the expiration date on your bottle of test strips.
3. If you have a machine that requires coding, check that the code on the bottle of strips matches your meter.
4. Prick your finger with the lancet or lancet pen and squeeze ("milk") your finger until you see a small drop of blood.
5. Move your finger next to the glucose strip so that the bead of blood is drawn into the absorbent strip. The strip will "grab" the droplet, so you won't have to press your finger directly to the strip.
6. Wait for the reading and record it in your log book.

Your health care team will determine the frequency of your testing, on the basis of the type of diabetes you have, your treatment regimen, and the stability of your glucose control.

surance plans cover at least a certain number of strips per month (say one hundred), but it's worth checking with your insurance company to be sure.

Over the past twenty-five years, glucose meters have become smaller, faster, and less complicated. Some models can store test results in memory or connect to a computer, in which case you can buy a software program to track glucose levels, diet, exercise, and insulin or medication over time. And for those with limited vision, some models have large display windows or the ability to speak to you.

Most meters follow the same procedure. You put the test strip in the meter, get a small drop of blood from a finger prick (or from an alternative site like the forearm), and touch the blood to the test strip. The meter measures how much glucose is present. Most often the blood sample is obtained by holding a pen-sized device called a lancet against the side of a fingertip (the side has fewer nerve endings than the tip) and pressing a button for a quick puncture. You do not need to

Checking your glucose
How to do a fingerstick

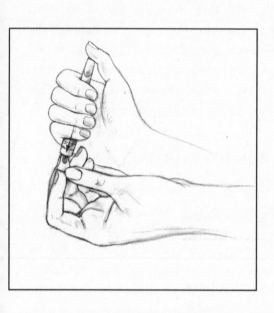

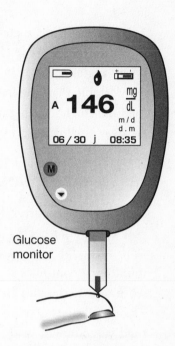

Glucose
monitor

A lancet penetrates the skin just enough to get a tiny drop of blood to test. Apply the drop of blood to the strip in the glucose meter, and in five to fifteen seconds your blood glucose level will appear on the display. See Appendix 4 for tips on how to choose a glucose meter.

use alcohol on your finger. The fingerstick may cause momentary, minimal discomfort. The meter will then display your glucose level, usually in five to fifteen seconds.

Keep a written log (a blood glucose diary) of glucose results and bring it to each medical appointment. In order to be most useful to your health care team, the log should contain the time of the tests, insulin dose if you take insulin, and other information regarding events that might affect glucose control (specific meals, parties, or exercise, for example). Although many meters can store and report the results of past tests, the meter's memory usually doesn't provide a day-to-day pattern of blood sugars. The blood glucose log is essential to understanding these patterns and determining if treatment needs to be adjusted.

At one time, meters required a "large, hanging drop of blood" to provide an accurate reading, but that's no longer the case. Some of the newer meters allow you to get blood from sites that are even less uncomfortable than the finger, such as the fleshy parts of the upper arm, the forearm, hand, thigh, or calf. After about a week or so, most people get over any initial squeamishness about pricking for blood.

LESS INVASIVE WAYS TO MONITOR GLUCOSE

Researchers are currently developing new ways to measure blood glucose using laser beams or light waves that do not involve pricking the skin. Although not yet accurate enough to take the place of current monitors, "continuous glucose monitoring systems" may one day be worn next to the skin and provide a constant read-out of glucose levels. The continuous glucose monitoring systems available now sample the fluid surrounding your skin cells with an indwelling micro-thin wire. The continuous monitors are not very accurate in the low range (less than 70 mg/dl). At this point, you still need to use your blood glucose meter three to four times a day to calibrate the continuous monitor. But manufacturers are currently refining these glucose sensors, which in the not-too-distant future should be able to continuously and accurately monitor the level of glucose. Someday, this technology will allow us to build an artificial pancreas that measures blood sugars continuously and delivers just the right amount of insulin to control blood sugar in the nondiabetic range.

OTHER MONITORING TESTS

As mentioned, self-monitoring of blood glucose has largely replaced urine testing. In fact, self-monitoring of blood glucose has revolutionized the care of type 1 diabetes, making intensive control and preven-

Glucose monitoring—Alternate sites for testing

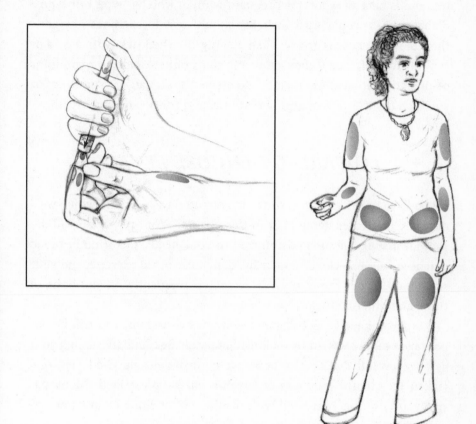

Some of the new meters allow you to get a drop of blood for monitoring from sites that are even less sensitive than the finger. The handheld lancet device (inset) is easy to use.

tion of complications possible. Although urine testing for sugar is still available, it is a poor, indirect measure of blood sugar levels and is rarely used. Urine testing *is* done, however, to detect ketones, the sign of a potentially life-threatening condition called ketoacidosis. Both urine and blood tests for ketones are available for home testing.

Ketone testing is an important part of monitoring type 1 diabetes, and is necessary for any pregnant woman who has type 1 or type 2 diabetes. All people with diabetes should test for ketones any time their blood glucose is greater than 300 mg/dl, when sick (with a cold or flu, for example), or if they show any signs of ketoacidosis. Symptoms of diabetic ketoacidosis include excessive thirst, nausea, vomiting, or stomach pains; labored, rapid breathing; and fruity-smelling breath.

LOWERING GLUCOSE LEVELS

If you have type 1 diabetes, you will be treated with insulin, which we'll describe in greater detail later in this chapter. Your physician will design an insulin regimen customized to your needs, factoring in blood glucose levels (checked frequently), diet, anticipated exercise, and your schedule. Insulin doses must be adjusted frequently on the basis of these and other factors.

If you have type 2 diabetes and are overweight, you will be encouraged to lose weight by making dietary changes and increasing your activity level. If that isn't sufficient to control your glucose levels, oral (taken by mouth) pills and/or insulin will be prescribed. Many patients are eventually treated with insulin, either alone or in combination with pills.

It used to be that this step-by-step approach for treating type 2 diabetes happened very slowly, and it would be years before medicines were added, and more years still before they were changed. By the time insulin was given, a person may have had diabetes for more than ten or even twenty years, at which point he or she would already have developed complications.

We now know that at least some of the disease's metabolic abnormalities, especially the decreasing secretion of insulin, can be reversed if glucose levels are normalized early enough in the disease process. Although some have been tempted to use the word "cure" in connection with this reversal, it is still not known if stabilization is per-

---

INSULIN USE IN TYPE 2 DIABETES

Your doctor may start you on insulin if:

- You have severe symptoms and/or very high glucose levels at the time of diagnosis.
- You experience diabetic ketoacidosis (DKA).
- You cannot achieve adequate glucose control with lifestyle changes and/ or oral medicines.
- You have persistent high blood glucose during pregnancy.

---

manent. But we do know enough to recommend that the slow, wait-and-see approach is no longer justified.

Insulin is the most potent drug in our glucose-lowering arsenal. But perhaps because it must be injected, it has in the past been saved as a last resort in treating type 2 diabetes. Diet is still the first approach taken to lower glucose levels. But don't be surprised if after a year or two of diet and pills, you are told you need insulin, the strongest medicine of all. Even after pills and/or insulin are added to your regimen, attention to lifestyle—diet and exercise—remain very important.

As shown in Table 7.2, there are five classes of oral medications currently used for treating type 2 diabetes. In addition, there are three types of injectable medications: insulin, pramlintide (Symilin), and exenatide (Byetta). Each class of drugs has a different way of controlling glucose levels.

A typical strategy for type 2 diabetes might be to start with metformin, which is the drug least likely to cause weight gain and one with few side effects. After a while, blood glucose monitoring may reveal that one drug alone is not enough to control your diabetes. Your physician may then add a sulfonylurea or go directly to insulin. Experience has shown us that certain drugs taken together produce a much greater beneficial effect than either alone. Your medical care team will determine which combination is best for you.

All five classes of oral drugs are currently approved for treating type 2 diabetes. Metformin and the drugs in the sulfonylurea class are

Table 7.2 Classes of oral medications and how they work

Type of oral medication	Target organ	Mechanism of action	Generic name (brand names)	Side effects				
				Low blood sugar	Weight gain	Digestive problems	Lactic acidosis	Liver function abnormalities
Sulfonylureas	Pancreas	Help the pancreas release more insulin	Glimepiride (Amaryl) Glipizide (Glucotrol, Glucotrol XL) Glyburide (Micronase, Diabeta, Glynase)	Yes	Yes	No	No	Very rare
Biguanides	Liver	Keep the liver from releasing too much sugar	Metformin (Glucophage, Glucophage XR)	No[a]	No	Yes	Very rare	No
Thiazolidinediones	Muscle cells, liver	Help cells use insulin better and lower insulin resistance	Pioglitazone (Actos) Rosiglitazone (Avandia)	No[a]	Yes[b]	No	No	Very rare
Meglitinides	Pancreas	Help pancreas release more insulin	Repaglinide (Prandin) Nateglinide (Starlix)	Yes	Yes	No	No	Very rare
Alpha-glucosidase Inhibitors	Small intestine	Slow the digestion of carbohydrates and prevent blood sugar from going too high after meals	Acarbose (Precose) Miglitol (Glyset)	No[a]	No	Common	No	Very rare

a. When used as the only therapy.
b. Edema (fluid retention) may occur.

BYETTA: THE NEW MED ON THE BLOCK

Byetta is a new class of FDA-approved medications for type 2 diabetes, classified as an "incretin mimetic." It's not an insulin, but it has to be injected. It is for those with type 2 diabetes who, despite taking various combinations of oral medications, still have high blood sugars. Incretin mimetics stimulate insulin production in response to high blood sugars, inhibit the release of glucagon from the liver after meals, and slow the absorption of food. Clinical studies have demonstrated a modest effect on hemoglobin A_{1c}, with a reduction of about 1 percent. In addition, this new class of drugs results in a modest degree of weight loss, about 3–5 pounds during the first six months. The major side effect is nausea.

those most commonly used alone, whereas the other drugs most often have supporting roles in therapy. In parentheses are the brand names for drugs that fall into each class. Table 7.3 details dosing ranges for the most common oral medications.

Increasingly, though, physicians are prescribing insulin in combination with one or more oral drugs. We believe that starting insulin early is an important strategy for achieving near-normal glucose control as early and as long as possible.

THE MIRACLE OF INSULIN

The successful use of insulin by Canadian researchers in 1921 to treat type 1 diabetes was followed shortly by its purification and widespread use. Hailed as a true medical miracle, insulin therapy put a halt to the uniform death sentence that accompanied the diagnosis of "juvenile-onset" diabetes. Insulin therapy saved the lives of those with what we now call type 1 diabetes.

Insulin is the only agent used to treat diabetes that occurs naturally in humans. Because insulin is a protein, it can't be given orally because it would be digested and never reach the bloodstream. Just about

Table 7.3   Dosing ranges for commonly used oral medications

Type of oral medication	Generic name (brand names)	Common dosages (mg) (total daily dose)
Sulfonylureas	Glimepiride (Amaryl)	1–8
	Glipizide (Glucotrol)	2.5–40
	Glipizide extended release (Glucotrol XL)	5–20
	Glyburide (Micronase, Diabeta)	1.25–20
	Glyburide (Glynase):	
	Regular form	1.25–20
	Micronized	0.75–12
Biguanides	Metformin (Glucophage)	1,000–3,000
	Metformin extended release (Glucophage XR)	500–2,000
	Glyburide/metformin (Glucovance)	1.25/250-20/2,000
Thiazolidinediones	Pioglitazone (Actos)	15–45
	Rosiglitazone (Avandia)	4–8
	Rosiglitazone/metformin (Avandamet)	4/1,000–8/2,000
Meglitinides	Repaglinide (Prandin)	1–16
	Nateglinide (Starlix)	180–360
Alpha-glucosidase inhibitors	Acarbose (Precose)	25–300
	Miglitol (Glyset)	25–300

Source: Adapted from Massachusetts Guidelines for Adult Diabetes Care, Diabetes Prevention and Control Program, Massachusetts Department of Public Health, 2005.

all the commercially available insulins now are genetically engineered as human insulin.

Insulin comes in a variety of preparations that differ according to how fast they take effect, when that effect is the greatest ("peak effect"), and how long they continue to work in the body ("duration" of effect). They are referred to as very rapid acting, regular or rapid acting, intermediate acting, or long acting. Table 7.4 describes some commonly used insulin preparations and how they work.

A woman with type 1 diabetes needs to take enough insulin at various times each day to keep blood glucose as close to nondiabetic levels as possible. To keep glucose from rising too high, particularly after meals, or falling too low, particularly during the night and between meals, she will require a combination of insulins or treatment with an insulin pump (described in the section called Pens, Patches, and Pumps later in this chapter, and in Appendix 7).

Insulin therapy for type 1 diabetes has two components—basal and bolus—designed to mimic what a person's own pancreas would do if she did not have diabetes. Basal insulin is meant to keep a stable insulin level throughout the day and night. For example, to cover the basal dose, you may take an intermediate-acting insulin in the morning and before bedtime, or perhaps one dose of long-acting insulin. Bolus insulin is designed to keep blood sugar levels under control— usually less than 180 mg/dl—at their peak after meals. This dose, administered before eating, is the one that may change at every meal, depending on various factors, such as meal size and composition and anticipated exercise after the meal. Most people with type 1 take either a very rapid–acting insulin ten to fifteen minutes before or a rapid-acting insulin thirty to forty-five minutes before each meal to prevent the large increase in glucose that otherwise occurs after food is absorbed.

The different types of insulin provide an opportunity for fine-tuning glucose levels, aided by frequent self-monitoring of blood glucose. With this information in hand, you are then also able to compensate for extra exercise, stress, illness, and the effects of your menstrual cycle. Premixed combinations of insulins are available commercially, but they are generally not recommended for type 1 diabetes.

Women with type 2 diabetes may also be prescribed insulin. But they may only need to take a basal insulin—for example, a long- or intermediate-acting insulin—once a day, before bedtime. The amount of insulin given, rather than the frequency, appears to be most crucial for keeping blood glucose under control with type 2 diabetes. Diabetes is a progressive disease, however, which is why self-monitoring is important. Someone with type 2 might need to add a bolus, premeal rapid-acting insulin at some point. Premixed insulins can be used with type 2 if prescribed by a physician. Table 7.5 lists some common problems with medications and offers some possible solutions.

Table 7.4 Insulin in action

Insulins vary as to when they start to work (onset of action), when the highest level of the insulin is in your bloodstream (peak), and how long they last in your body (duration). This table lists the different types of insulin available.

Type of insulin Brand name (generic)	Appearance of insulin	Onset of action	Peak	Duration of action	Recommendations
Very rapid acting Humalog (lispro) Novolog (aspart) Apidra (glulysine)	Clear	5–15 minutes	1–2 hours	4–6 hours	Because these insulins work so quickly, you need to eat within 10–15 minutes after taking them. The amount you take will often be based on your blood sugar level, meal size and carbohydrate content, and anticipated exercise
Rapid acting Humulin R (human regular) Novolin R (human regular) Velosulin BR (human regular)	Clear	30–60 minutes	2–3 hours	6–8 hours	Usually injected 1/2 hour before meals
Intermediate acting Humulin N (NPH, human isophane suspension) Novolin N (NPH, human isophane suspension)	Cloudy	1–3 hours	4–8 hours	10–16 hours	Often given before breakfast and/or dinner or bedtime
Long acting Lantus (recombinant human analog, glargine) Levemir (Detimer)	Clear	2 hours	None	24–30 hours Up to 24 hours	Cannot be mixed with other insulins in same syringe

Mixtures

	Onset	Peak	Duration
Humulin 70/30			
(70 percent NPH, human isophane suspension, and	1–3 hours	4–8 hours	12–14 hours
30 percent human regular)	30–60 minutes	2–3 hours	6–8 hours
Novolin 70/30			
(70 percent NPH, human isophane suspension, and	1–3 hours	4–8 hours	12–14 hours
30 percent human regular)	30–60 minutes	2–3 hours	6–8 hours
Humalog Mix 75/25			
(75 percent insulin lispro protamine suspension [NPH-like] and	15 minutes	4–8 hours	12–14 hours
25 percent insulin lispro)	5–15 minutes	1–2 hours	4–6 hours
Novolog Mix 70/30			
(70 percent NPH human isophane suspension and	15 minutes	4–8 hours	12–14 hours
30 percent insulin aspart)	5–15 minutes	1–2 hours	4–6 hours

Source: Adapted from Kathy Hurxthal, *An Introduction to Diabetes* (Diabetes Center, Massachusetts General Hospital, 2002).

Table 7.5   Common problems with medications

Problem	Solution
Too expensive	Discuss less expensive medications with your medical provider.
Easy to mix up	Label everything and use a pill box.
Running out of medication	Note when refills are done.
Forgetting to take pills —interruptions in daily routine —work schedule	Set up a schedule that is easy to remember. Ask your medical team which medications can be taken together. Discuss how to simplify timing of medications.
Fear of side effects	Know the side effects and talk to your medical provider if you notice any symptoms.

METHOD OF INJECTION

If you're like most people, you may cringe at the idea of injecting yourself with a syringe. Most people envision the long, painful needles used for vaccinations. The new insulin syringe needles are very, very thin and virtually pain-free. The health benefits of insulin therapy are well worth getting over any initial reluctance or fears. After some practice, most people master the technique quite easily. And if you are already accustomed to pricking your finger to self-monitor blood glucose, you'll find that injection hurts even less.

Your diabetes nurse educator will help you feel more comfortable about injections and teach you how to do them properly. You pinch a bit of skin at the site of injection, then insert the syringe at a correct angle before pushing down on the plunger to inject the insulin. You can practice by filling one of your syringes with air or water and injecting it into an orange. Studies have found that cleaning the skin with alcohol before the injection, as was once routinely advised, may not be necessary. You can even inject through clothing without affecting the absorption of the insulin. The sites of injection should be rotated so your skin doesn't get irritated. Common sites include the abdomen (where absorption is the quickest), the arm, and the thighs and buttocks (the sites where absorption is the slowest).

Insulin injection sites

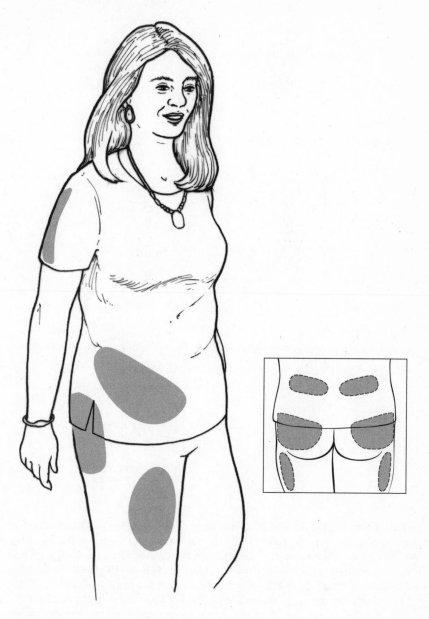

The shaded areas are the common injection sites, which should be rotated to avoid skin irritation.

Preparing the injection

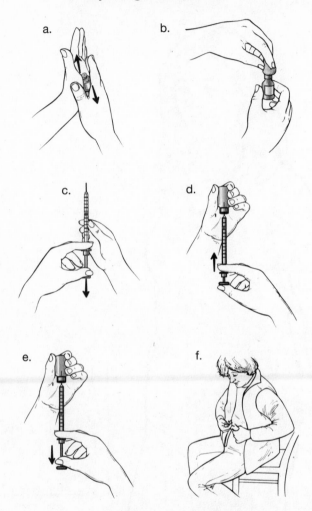

(a) First, gently roll the insulin vial in the palms of your hands to make sure it is mixed evenly. (b) Wipe the rubber lid of the vial with cotton dipped in alcohol or an alcohol wipe. (c) Before putting the needle into the vial, withdraw the syringe plunger to the correct amount of insulin, drawing air into it. (d) Insert the needle through the stopper on the insulin bottle and push the plunger to inject the air into the vial. (e) Then, without removing the needle from the vial, draw the correct amount of insulin into the syringe. Check for air bubbles and tap the side of the syringe's barrel if you see any. Doublecheck that you have the right amount of insulin before removing the needle. (f) Pinch a bit of skin and insert the syringe at a correct angle before pushing down on the plunger to inject the insulin. Rotate the site of injection from the abdomen, arms, thighs, and buttocks.

You will also learn the proper technique for filling the syringe with insulin. First, check the label to make sure you are using the correct type of insulin. Then gently roll the insulin vial or insulin pen in the palms of your hands (or shake gently) to make sure it is mixed evenly. This step is not necessary for all types of insulin, but it's a good habit to get into.

Before putting the needle into the vial, withdraw the syringe plunger to the correct amount of insulin, drawing air into the syringe. Insert the needle through the stopper on the insulin bottle and push the plunger to inject the air into the vial. Then, without removing the needle from the vial, draw the correct amount of insulin into the syringe. Check for air bubbles; if there are any, hold the syringe with the needle pointing up and flick the side of it once or twice. Air bubbles take up space, and you want to make sure you get the proper dose of insulin.

Insulin is a potent medication, so be sure to measure precisely how much you give yourself. It's like baking, where following the recipe exactly is critical to the final product. Too much or too little will affect your blood sugar levels.

Be aware, too, that it is a common error to confuse the dosages for two different kinds of insulin. You might grab the vial of a rapid-acting insulin, thinking it is an intermediate-acting one, and give yourself the wrong dose. When you realize your mistake, follow the procedure to avoid hypoglycemia (see page 110). At one time you could tell rapid-acting (clear) and intermediate-acting (cloudy) insulins by their appearance. But now there's glargine, a twenty-four-hour insulin that is clear, so this distinction is no longer always true.

Here are some other insulin tips:

→ Activities that increase your skin temperature and local blood flow, for example, running, may increase the rate of insulin absorption by the exercising limb. In addition, sauna, hot baths, and massage of the injection site will increase the rate at which the insulin is absorbed.

→ Vials of insulin should be refrigerated but never frozen; insulin is also relatively stable at room temperature.

➡ Don't use insulin after its expiration date. It may also lose some of its strength if the bottle has been used for more than a month, particularly if it was not refrigerated.

➡ In the United States, insulin is most often found in a concentration of 100 units/ml (called U-100) and, for rare occasions when large doses are necessary, as 500 units/ml (U-500). Travelers should be aware that insulin is sometimes found in a strength of U-40 in other countries; if you must use U-40, be sure to use a syringe designated for U-40.

➡ Different types of insulin (for example, rapid-acting and intermediate-acting) are often mixed immediately before injection to create the right profile of insulin activity for you. You'll need to pay special attention to how you mix insulins (see Appendix 5 for directions).

➡ Reuse of syringes is safe, but syringes should never be shared. Repeated use (more than three or four times) may dull the needle and cause a little more discomfort.

➡ Used syringes should be disposed of properly. Some communities have disposal programs available. If not, before they are discarded used "sharps" should be put in some kind of container that cannot be punctured. See Appendix 6 for how to dispose of syringes.

Pens, Patches, and Pumps

There are several alternative methods for injecting or "delivering" insulin. Insulin pens, for example, are prefilled with about 300 units of insulin. You set a dial to the amount of insulin you need, attach a needle tip and, with the push of a button, inject the insulin into the skin as you would with a syringe. The needle is replaced after each injection, as is the insulin cartridge when it is empty, although some pens are completely disposable after they are empty. Insulin pens are convenient to carry and use. But as with any insulin, pens should not be left in a hot car, or anywhere too hot or too cold.

High-pressure jet injectors force a tiny stream of insulin mixed with air through the skin. These devices don't puncture the skin but can bruise it if they are not used correctly. Some people find they are actually more painful than needles. They are also expensive, require a lot of care, and may not be covered by your health insurance.

Inhaled insulin and a delivery system were approved by the FDA in 2006. The device works much like a larger version of an asthma inhaler: you breathe in a rapid-acting insulin by mouth to the lungs, where it can pass into the bloodstream. Only a very small amount (about 10 percent) actually reaches the bloodstream, however, which means that much larger amounts of insulin (about ten times as much as an injection) are necessary to get an effective dose. The long-term effects on the lungs are not yet known, though no clinically significant adverse effects have been seen after as long as two years of use. This device is extremely appealing to many patients, especially those with type 1 diabetes who need to take numerous doses of insulin each day.

Insulin patches and even oral insulins are also being explored as a means of delivering insulin. Insulin does not pass through the skin or intestines easily, however, and these delivery routes remain experimental.

For those with type 1 diabetes, the insulin pump is an attractive alternative that has been available since the 1970s. Its technology has dramatically improved since then. About the size of a beeper or cell phone, the pump is worn on a belt or carried in a pocket. It delivers insulin through very thin tubing that is inserted under the skin, usually in the abdomen, with a thin needle. A constant flow of very-rapid or rapid-acting insulin provides the basal, and the pump-user tells the pump how much to give as a bolus dose before meals.

The pump does not do everything, however; pump-users still need to measure blood sugar frequently so they can instruct the pump correctly. Some meters help guide the patient in the choice of doses, on the basis of information that has been programmed into the meter. Like all those with type 1 diabetes, pump users should count carbohydrates and closely monitor their food intake. For someone motivated to learn to operate it, the pump can provide an added level of control and even flexibility, since adjusting insulin and giving frequent doses of insulin may be easier for them.

In the future, continuous glucose monitors paired with insulin pumps will be "smart" enough to do it all for you, as close to an artificial pancreas as anyone can imagine.

MEDICAL NUTRITION THERAPY

For most people with diabetes, diet cannot be the sole treatment, but it is still a critical component of disease management. Although the universal "diabetic diet" is a thing of the past, there are general goals for meal planning and healthful eating that apply to all women with diabetes. You will also need to develop specific goals tailored to your individual needs and to the type of diabetes you have.

Everyone, with or without diabetes, can improve her health by making better food choices and increasing physical activity. With diabetes, it becomes even more important to eat the right amounts of the three major nutrients—protein, carbohydrates, and fats—and to avoid large fluctuations in the amount you eat from day to day. This will help to keep blood glucose levels stable and as close to the nondiabetic range as possible to prevent or reduce the risk of complications. It will also help keep your lipid profile and blood pressure in a range that will reduce the likelihood of cardiovascular disease and stroke. If you are overweight or obese, as are most women with type 2 diabetes, dietary changes can result in weight loss—and even modest losses lead to big gains in health. The same is true for women with prediabetes; as high-quality clinical trials have shown, healthy lifestyle changes can prevent diabetes from developing in the first place (see Chapter 3).

For women with type 1 diabetes, diet takes on an additional role. What you eat is integral to deciding how much insulin you should take. Your bolus dose of insulin before meals is based on your level of glucose and what you plan to eat. Carbohydrates have the greatest effect on blood glucose because they are broken down into sugar. Some carbohydrates, such as table sugar, have an almost immediate effect on blood sugar levels, while others must be broken down in the intestine and are absorbed more slowly. In general, the more fiber in a food, the slower the absorption of the carbohydrate. By counting the grams of carbohydrates you will be eating, and understanding how different carbohydrates are absorbed, you can figure out more precisely how much insulin you will need. We'll discuss how to count carbs later in this chapter.

For women with type 2 diabetes, cutting calories (usually by reducing fat content), reducing salt, and eating more fiber are often recommended. Since type 2 diabetes is usually associated with being overweight or obese, weight loss is one of the most important goals to strive for. A modest weight loss of 7 to 10 percent of your body weight (your weight multiplied by .07 to .10) can prevent type 2 diabetes and improve elevated glucose levels if you already have diabetes. This is your incentive, particularly if you've recently been diagnosed with type 2 diabetes. You can reverse the disease process in its early stages and never need any medications at all if you lose weight and *keep it off.* It is never too late, however, to gain some benefit from weight loss.

In most parts of the country, the diabetes team will include a dietitian who will devise a medical nutrition plan, starting with an analysis of what you're eating now. You will set goals and receive guidance on how to reach them. Your progress will be monitored through periodic checks of HgbA$_{1c}$, lipids, blood pressure, and weight loss. The food you will be encouraged to eat will be good for everyone else in your family, too. The emphasis will be on limiting saturated fats, cholesterol, and sweets, and eating more fruits, vegetables, and whole grains. But your meal plan will also take into account your preferences, be it the ethnic foods you're accustomed to, the tastes you enjoy, or the timing of your meals.

The general goals of medical nutrition therapy are to

- ➡ keep blood glucose levels as close to the nondiabetic range as possible, and lower lipid and blood pressure levels to reduce the risk of vascular diseases;
- ➡ provide enough calories and activity to better balance "calories in" (what we eat) with "calories out" (what's burned up for energy), and eat at consistent times during the day;
- ➡ target healthy amounts of key nutrients (carbohydrates, fat, protein) for each meal; if you take insulin, keep the intake of carbohydrates

fairly consistent from day to day. When your carbohydrate intake varies, you'll need to know how to adjust insulin doses to keep glucose levels stable and in an acceptable range;

➡ modify nutrients and lifestyle factors to promote long-term health and, in particular, to help you achieve and maintain a healthier weight.

NUTRITIONAL GUIDELINES

- 45–65 percent of your daily calories should come from carbohydrates; 15–20 percent from protein (unless you have kidney disease); 20–30 percent from fat (less than 10 percent from saturated fat and mostly mono- and polyunsaturated fats). In addition, you should get at least 20–35 grams of fiber each day.

- For weight loss, a goal of one pound every one to two weeks is ideal, accomplished by reducing the number of calories you consume by 250 to 500 per day. Total calories should not be less than 1,000–1,200 for women (1,200–1,600 for men).

- A target of 60–90 minutes of moderately intense physical activity is encouraged most days of the week, with a minimum of 150–175 minutes per week. This should include cardiovascular, stretching, and resistance exercises.

Source: Adapted from the American Diabetes Association (Position Statement). Standards of Care for Patients with Diabetes. *Diabetes Care,* 29 (51) (2006).

NUTRIENTS WE NEED

Proteins, carbohydrates, and fats are all essential for a healthy body to function. Most Americans consume more than enough of each of these nutrients. Generally, it is not advisable to cut way down on any one of these nutrients in an attempt to lose weight. Eating a variety of foods (see the food pyramids on pages 56–57) is key to a nutrition plan you can stick with. If you feel deprived, you probably won't succeed long term with any program.

All three of these nutrients contain calories, but because fat holds much less water, it has two time more calories by weight than

Food portions
Everything in moderation

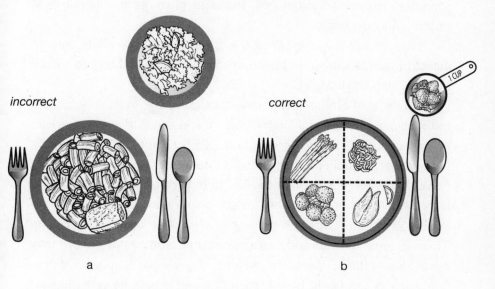

(a) A common mistake is to load your plate. Bigger portions mean more calories taken in. (b) Controlling the size of food portions and eating a balanced diet are key to a healthy lifestyle.

carbohydrates and proteins. No more than 30 percent of your daily calories should come from fats (and less than 10 percent of that amount should come from saturated fats). Your body needs fat for energy, making certain hormones, regulating blood pressure, and keeping your skin and hair healthy. But there can be too much of even a good thing. If we eat more fat (or any of the food groups) than we need, the excess calories get stored in fat cells, and over time we get fatter.

Though fats in general should be limited, some are healthier than others. The general rule of thumb is that saturated fats (typically fats that come from animal versus plant products) promote the formation of artery-clogging fatty deposits. Saturated fats and trans fatty acids—found in snack foods, baked products, and fried chicken—are the worst fats because they tend to increase the LDL blood cholesterol, the cholesterol that is linked to heart disease. Unsaturated fats are preferable. The unsaturated, "good" fats are found in avocados, oils (olive, canola, peanut), peanut butter, and nuts (almonds, cashews, hazelnuts, peanuts). Monounsaturated fats, found in olive oil and certain fish, promote healthy hearts.

In Chapter 3 we explained the differences between fats, how to detect hidden fats in foods, how to read food labels, and how to reduce the "bad" fats in your diet.

Sources of protein include meat, chicken, fish, milk, cheese, eggs, tofu, peanuts, lentils, chick peas, yogurt, and soy. A typical American consumes about 15 to 20 percent of her daily calories as protein, more than enough to fulfill the critical role proteins play in all biological processes in the body. You don't need to limit protein intake because you have diabetes (protein does not affect blood glucose), unless you are getting much more than 20 percent of your daily calories as protein. There is some indication that such excessive amounts of protein may contribute to the development of kidney disease. Many sources of protein, such as meats, do have hidden fats and should be eaten in moderation. Certain fish—salmon, tuna, and sardines—by contrast, have omega-3 fats, which are heart-healthy.

Recommendations for how many carbohydrates overweight or obese people with diabetes should have each day range widely from very low amounts in the Atkins diet to very high amounts in the Pritikin and Ornish diets (see Chapter 3). However, most people with diabetes should get between 45 and 55 percent of their total intake from carbohydrates. The position taken by the American Diabetes Association's panel of experts is that carbohydrates and monounsaturated fat (the good kind) together should provide 60 to 70 percent of the diabetic diet.

As with fats, not all carbohydrates are equally healthful. Some carbohydrates (vegetables and fruits) are loaded with valuable nutrients, but others (soda) are laden with calories that contribute nothing our bodies need to survive. The solution is not to banish all carbohydrates but to make healthy choices.

THE IMPORTANCE OF CALCIUM

A multivitamin usually ensures you're getting sufficient vitamins and minerals, but the other supplement women really should take is calcium, ideally with vitamin D to aid absorption. (Folate, taken to prevent birth defects at least three months before and during pregnancy, is also important.)

Women need at least 1,200–1,500 mg of calcium to reduce bone loss (osteoporosis), especially after menopause. Since much of the calcium we ingest is not absorbed, most women do not get this much. Taking a 500 mg supplement twice or more daily can improve absorption.

Are you getting enough calcium? Dietary sources of calcium include:

- Milk and dairy products—8 ounces of milk (fat free, low fat, or whole) has 300 mg, 2 ounces of American cheese has 350 mg, 1 ounce of cheddar cheese has 204 mg, plain fat-free yogurt has 450 mg, yogurt with fruit has 315 mg.

- Dark green, leafy vegetables—one cup of broccoli has 90 mg, 1/2 cup of spinach has 122 mg.

- Foods with calcium added—8 ounces of orange juice fortified with calcium has 300 mg, 1/2 cup of fat-free frozen yogurt has 450 mg.

- Nuts and grains—1 ounce roasted almonds has 80 mg, 1 slice of bread (white or wheat) has 30 mg.

Carbohydrates are found in fruit; dairy products like milk and yogurt; grains and grain products, like bread, cereal, rice, and pasta; and vegetables. Fruits and vegetables are loaded with vitamins A and C and other vitamins and minerals we need; dairy products are too, including calcium and to a certain extent vitamin D, which are critical to the prevention of bone-thinning disease in women.

Sugars are also carbohydrates and are found in sweets like cake, soda, candy, honey, and jelly. These foods provide calories but little else of nutritional value. More important, they are rapidly absorbed and, in people with diabetes, quickly raise blood sugars to high levels. It is no longer considered necessary to eliminate sugar from your diet, as long as you count it as a carbohydrate and adjust any insulin you may take accordingly. But it is important to learn how to satisfy your sweet

COMMON FORMS OF SUGAR FOUND ON FOOD LABELS

- Sugar
- Brown sugar
- Dextrose
- Fructose
- Corn syrup
- Honey
- Maple syrup
- Sucrose
- Confectioners' sugar
- Malt, maltose
- High-fructose corn syrup
- Molasses
- Turbinado sugar (dark brown raw sugar from sugar cane)

tooth without always turning to high-calorie, low-nutrition sweets. One way to do this, for example, is to reduce the amount of sugar called for in recipes or to use sugar-free or no-calorie sweeteners. (But be sure to read the labels carefully when buying sugar-free products. Often they have more fat or other sugar substitutes.)

Most of the carbohydrates you consume should be whole-grain, high-fiber foods. Fiber comes only from plant sources and is not digested, so it contributes no calories. But it does have benefits, particularly for people with diabetes. Generally, fiber is classified as soluble and insoluble. Insoluble fibers—found in whole-grain breads, whole-grain cereals, wheat bran, legumes (peas and beans), cabbage, beets, cauliflower, and brussel sprouts—increase the speed that food moves through your gastrointestinal system. As a result, insoluble fibers don't slow the rise in blood glucose very much.

Soluble fibers, by contrast, slow the rise in blood glucose after a meal, thus lowering the amount of insulin needed. They also help

SOURCES OF FIBER (3 GRAMS OR MORE PER SERVING)

Baked apple (1 = 5 grams)

Raspberries (1/2 cup = 4.5 grams)

Pear with skin (1 medium = 4 grams)

Raw strawberries (1 cup = 3.5 grams)

Cooked greens (1 cup = 4 grams)

Cooked green peas (1/2 cup = 4 grams)

Baked potato with skin (1 medium = 5 grams)

Peanuts (1/4 cup = 4.5 grams)

Lentils (2/3 cup = 4.5 grams)

Whole-wheat bread (2 slices = 4 grams)

For more information, see the American Dietetic Association at www.eatright.org.

lower cholesterol levels. Sources of soluble fiber are dried peas and beans, apples, carrots, potatoes, and oats. If you have type 1 diabetes, understanding how this form of fiber works is useful in planning the doses of insulin you'll need.

For those with type 2 diabetes, the effect of fiber in slowing absorption of sugar may be just what you need. In type 2 diabetes, often there is not enough insulin released during the first half-hour after a meal to override insulin resistance. If the rise in blood glucose is slowed by soluble fiber–containing foods, the pancreas has more time to catch up.

Ideally, everyone should get twenty to thirty-five grams of fiber each day—about twice the amount most Americans currently consume. You can do that by eating more unrefined food products. The refining process used to make white flour, for example, removes almost all the fiber from grains. The same thing happens to white rice during the refining process, which is why brown rice is a healthier choice. You can also boost your fiber intake by eating the skins of potatoes and fruits, since the skins contain a lot of fiber. Fruits are always preferable to fruit juice, in which fiber has been removed. An added bonus of eating more fiber is that you will feel more full—and less likely to overeat.

COUNTING CARBS AND OTHER APPROACHES TO MEAL PLANNING

For the vast majority of women with type 2 diabetes, lifestyle change focuses on decreasing fat, keeping portions small and calories down, and increasing activity. We go into great detail on how to accomplish these goals in Chapter 3. These same strategies for preventing diabetes are also useful if you've been diagnosed with the disease.

For most women it is sufficient to be conscious of carbohydrates, to eat the healthier ones, and to keep the amounts eaten pretty consistent throughout the day. But people with type 1 diabetes, usually because they are intensively controlling their blood glucose levels, turn to more advanced methods of accounting for the effects of the carbohydrates they eat on their blood glucose levels.

In the past, meal planning was done by "meal exchange" lists. As part of your meal plan, your dietitian would recommend the number of servings from each food group (carbohydrate, fat, protein) that you should include in each meal to meet your goal in calories for that day. Within each food group were subcategories (under carbohydrates, for example, would be starch, milk, fruit, and vegetables). Established portions of foods within these subcategories could be exchanged to make up a meal.

Exchange lists are still used, but today it is more common to "count carbs," that is, to count the number of grams of carbohydrates in a given meal, making sure that you don't exceed your goal for that meal and that day. Carb counting entails reading food labels, looking up amounts of carbohydrates found in particular foods, and measuring portions. This meal-planning approach tends to be less complicated

---

APPROACHES TO ADJUSTING CARBOHYDRATES IN YOUR DIET

Basic approach (for those with type 2 diabetes who are not on insulin)

• Eat consistent amounts of carbohydrates at meals and snack time.

• Seek guidance from a certified nutritionist or weight-loss program if you are trying to lose weight.

Carbohydrate counting (usually for those with type 1 diabetes)

• Adjust your insulin dose to match your carbohydrate intake (count grams of carbohydrates).

• To ensure that you are getting an accurate dose of insulin, learn how to estimate food portions and know how many carbohydrates are in each portion.

• Meet with a certified nutritionist or attend diabetes education classes to learn the nuances of carbohydrate counting.

---

than "meal exchanges" because the focus is on one nutrient. It also allows for greater flexibility in food choices. In Appendix 2, we list some carbohydrate counts for common foods.

A more elaborate way of accounting for carbs is to add them up according to their "glycemic index." This method is based on the fact that carbohydrates vary in their effects on blood sugar. The glycemic index is a ranking of carbs from 0 to 100: the lower numbers below 55 are assigned to foods that are digested slowly and don't cause a spike in blood glucose; and the high numbers, above 70, are for those that do. Some studies have shown benefits, in terms of glucose and lipid control, of following diets with low glycemic indexes for those with either type 1 or type 2 diabetes. Other studies are less convincing.

It is important to note, however, that the index takes into account the effect but not the amount of a particular carbohydrate. For example, a raw carrot has a high glycemic index rating of 131, but that's because the glycemic effect is calculated based on a 50 gram serving of each carbohydrate, which for carrots would be like eating 1 1/2 pounds. So some advocates have sensibly suggested that the

---

CARBOHYDRATES AND THE GLYCEMIC INDEX

Low glycemic index (usually high-fiber foods)

- High-fiber fruits and vegetables
- Bran cereals
- Soy beans
- Chick peas, kidney beans, black beans, red lentils, and pinto beans

Medium glycemic index

- Pearled barley
- Brown rice
- Oatmeal
- Bulgur
- Rice cakes
- Whole-grain breads and pasta
- No-sugar added fruit juices

High glycemic index

- Baked potato
- French fries
- Refined cereal products
- Sugar-sweetened beverages
- Candy
- Couscous
- White rice, pasta, and bread
- Bagels

Source: Adapted from K. Foster-Powell, S. H. Holt, and J. C. Brand-Miller, "International Table of Glycemic Index and Glycemic Load Values: 2002," *American Journal of Clinical Nutrition* 76 (2002): 5–56.

---

index be further refined to include the calculation of "glycemic load," multiplication of the glycemic index times the quantity.

Although the jury is still out on the health benefits of meal planning based on the glycemic index, it is clear that careful monitoring of carbohydrates does guide people toward healthier eating. The low index/load foods point consumers to a strategy that is generally recommended: eat healthy carbs, including fiber-rich fruits, vegetables, and whole-grain foods, along with adequate protein and healthy fats.

WEIGHT CONTROL

As part of your medical nutrition plan you may be encouraged to set a goal for reducing the number of calories you consume and increasing the number you expend through physical activity. In Chapter 3 we described strategies for preventing diabetes by regaining better balance of "calories in/calories out." These same strategies apply to those who already have diabetes. You've got equally strong incentives to make a change.

The late comedian Jackie Gleason once said: "The second day of a diet is always easier than the first. By the second day, you're off it."

We're not talking about dieting in the sense of futilely trying one fad diet after another in hopes it will be the one that works. We're talking about making changes in your lifestyle that you can live with day in and day out for the rest of your life. There are ways to lose weight, albeit slowly, without depriving yourself of food variety and taste to the point that you are doomed not to stick with the program for long.

Your initial weight-loss goal will probably be based on 7 to 10 percent of your current weight. Your dietitian will help you calculate how many calories you have been consuming and how many you need to cut out each day for six months to reach that goal. The goal will entail cutting out something like 400 calories a day to lose about one pound every ten days. Current evidence favors accomplishing this reduction of calories by limiting fats from your diet and increasing daily exercise. But certainly your successes and failures in dieting in the past will be taken into account as you and your dietitian search for an approach that will work for you. Incorporating increased activity levels into your new lifestyle will help rebalance your calories in and calories out.

Keeping weight off is unquestionably difficult, more difficult than losing the weight in the first place. Many obese people, for example, have their genes stacked against them. Genetic factors involved in the regulation of appetite and body weight appear to predispose some people to obesity. But the evidence shows that weight loss can be maintained if we make some commonsense changes:

→ Downsize portions, especially at dinner.
→ Restrict fat, sugar, and high-calorie foods and beverages.
→ Eat more slowly.
→ Do not skip breakfast (spread calories throughout the day).
→ Reduce the emotional reasons for overeating (see Chapter 6).
→ Become more active by planning physical activity such as walking, swimming, or yoga and increasing everyday activities, such as using the stairs instead of an elevator.

Weight-loss medications may be helpful for some people, but they should be used only in addition to these lifestyle strategies and under the direction of your health care team. Medications only work as long as they are taken.

We will cover the surgical options for treating obesity in the next chapter. The risks of these procedures dictate that they should be considered only in severely obese individuals, defined as those with a BMI greater than 40, or for those with diabetes, a BMI greater than 35.

KEEP MOVING

You need to restrict your food intake to lose weight. Exercise alone won't help you with that. But it's a perfect partner with dietary changes because the more you move, the more calories you burn up. Exercise is key to maintaining weight loss. Exercise also improves insulin sensitivity—one of the major abnormalities of type 2 diabetes—ensuring that the insulin released or given will be maximally effective. Regular exercise probably also reduces the risk of cardiovascular disease and in general makes you feel good.

Table 7.6 Calories burned in thirty minutes of activity

Activity	Calories burned for 150 lb. person
Bicycling 10–12 mph	204
Gardening	170
Tennis	238
Jogging	238
Swimming leisurely	200
Walking 3 mph	119
Golf (only if you walk the course)	187
Ice skating	235
Sitting quietly	34
Standing	68

Source: Adapted from B. E. Ainsworth, et al., "Medicine and Science in Sports and Exercise," *Journal of the American College of Sports Medicine* 25 (1993): 71–80.

As discussed in Chapter 3, everything that gets you off the couch counts as activity, from walking from your car to the store, gardening, and housework, to chasing after a toddler. But added benefits come from more sustained aerobic activity, such as exercise classes, walking, running, or biking. You can reap enormous benefit from moderate activity such as walking for twenty to thirty minutes three to five times a week (see Table 7.6). Weight-resistance training adds other benefits, increasing muscle mass and slowing the loss of bone mass that is associated with aging and puts women at higher risk for osteoporosis.

Women with type 1 diabetes need to plan for their exercise so they can adjust the amount of insulin they take. Alternatively, they need to compensate for physical activity by eating an additional carbohydrate. Someone with type 2 diabetes usually doesn't have to do this.

All women with diabetes should check with their health care team before starting a new exercise program. The presence of micro- or macrovascular complications may mean that certain activities won't be recommended for you. You may also have to take precautions to prevent foot problems (especially with high-impact activities like jogging), for example, by using foot padding, special socks to prevent blisters, and proper footwear. But there is a safe activity for everyone.

EXERCISE TIPS

- Remember that anything that gets you moving counts. Pick up the pace of your usual activities, like housecleaning, gardening, or walking the dog.
- Wear appropriate foot gear.
- Replenish lost fluids by drinking water before and after exercise.
- Stretch before exercising.
- Exercise with a friend or family member.
- Try to schedule exercise at the same time each day. Write it down on your calendar.
- Gradually build up time, starting with as little as ten minutes a day.
- If you are on insulin therapy: test your blood sugar before and after exercise; adjust medications, if necessary; have a snack if your blood glucose is less than 100.
- Check with your health care team before starting a new exercise program.

DETERMINING A TARGET HEART RATE FOR EXERCISE

1. Calculate your maximum heart rate by subtracting your age from 220.
2. Multiple this number by 0.7 for a target exercise heart rate of 70 percent of your maximum heart rate.
3. After you exercise for a couple of months, you can increase your heart rate to 85 percent of your maximum heart rate.
4. Check with your physician. She may adjust the target rate based on the presence of heart disease or the results of an exercise tolerance test.

Checking your pulse

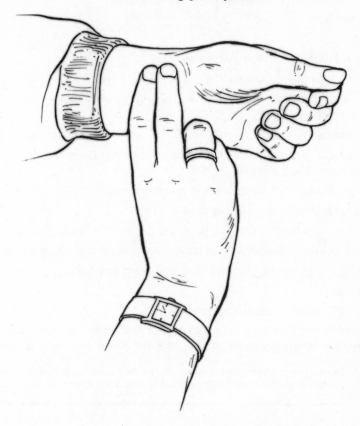

You want to find an aerobic activity that will make your heart beat faster but not too fast. To check your heartbeat, place two fingers (not the thumb, which has its own pulse) on your wrist just below the thumb. Count the number of throbs you feel in ten seconds, and multiply that figure by six to compute your heartbeats per minute. Is this within the target range for your age?

To get your maximum heart rate, subtract your age from 220. The target training zone is about 70 to 85 percent of your maximum heart rate. For example, if you are age 50, then 220 − 50 = 170, your maximum heart rate. Your target range is 170 × .70 = 119 and 170 × .85 = 145 beats per minute.

SAFETY GUIDELINES FOR EXERCISE

Before exercise

- Warm up

If you take insulin or a sulfonylurea

- Check your blood glucose. If it's below 100, have a snack.
- Ask your doctor whether you should change your dosage before exercising.

During exercise

- Wear your medical identification bracelet or other ID, which should note if you have heart disease.
- Increase intensity and duration of exercise slowly.

If you take insulin or a sulfonylurea

- Always carry food or glucose tablets to be ready to treat hypoglycemia.
- If exercising for more than one hour, check your blood glucose regularly.
- You may need to eat snacks before you finish exercising.

After exercise

If you take insulin or a sulfonylurea

- Check to see how exercise affected your blood glucose level. Low blood sugar levels may occur for as long as 6–12 hours after vigorous exercise.

Source: Adapted from "What I Need to Know about Physical Activity and Diabetes," National Diabetes Information Clearinghouse (http://diabetes.niddk.nih.gov/dm/pubs/physical_ez/index.htm).

MANAGING DIABETIC COMPLICATIONS

Intensive control of blood glucose is a powerful way to prevent the development of the medical complications that can result from diabetes. The earlier in the disease process you can get your blood glucose down and the longer it stays down, the better off you will be. Even when you've started to develop complications, targeting blood glucose levels is a way to slow progression of the various disease processes affecting the eyes, nervous system, and kidneys.

Diabetes is also accompanied by a major increased risk of plaque-clogging diseases of the large blood vessels to the heart, brain, and

BUILDING A PARTNERSHIP WITH YOUR MEDICAL TEAM

- Schedule an appointment for every three to six months.
- Prepare for your medical visit:

  –Bring your diabetes log or diary with a record of glucose monitoring readings, what you ate, when you exercised, and your insulin doses.

  –Bring your list of medications and note which ones need to be refilled.

  –Write down your questions and concerns, such as:

  - Has anything happened in your life that may be affecting your diabetes?
  - What times of day do you feel best (worst)?
  - Have you been gaining (losing) weight?
  - How often do you exercise?
  - Have you had any recent episodes of hypoglycemia? If so, have they appeared in a pattern, such as at a specific time of day? Was there an obvious cause (such as delay of medications)?

  –Ask a family member to come with you for support.

  –If you are non–English-speaking, ask your medical provider to arrange for an interpreter.

peripheral vascular system (the extremities). There's a cascade effect leading from obesity to type 2 diabetes to heart disease and stroke. In Chapter 4 we discussed in detail the various complications and how to prevent or treat them. Here's a brief reminder:

- → reduce and maintain HgbA$_{1c}$ less than 7 percent
- → reduce blood pressure to less than 130/80 mmHg
- → reduce LDL to less than 100 mg/dl; lower triglycerides to less than 150 mg/dl; raise HDL above 50 mg
- → quit cigarette smoking if you smoke
- → lose weight if you're overweight, and exercise most days of the week
- → take a low-dose of aspirin daily
- → schedule yearly eye exams
- → schedule yearly kidney function tests

YOUR COMPREHENSIVE DIABETES EVALUATION

Although you may visit a member of your diabetes care team every three to six months, you can expect a comprehensive evaluation of how you're doing annually. This will include:

- Medical history and review of current treatment
- Eating patterns and nutritional status
- Details of previous diabetes treatment and educational programs
- Assessment of personal health attitudes and beliefs; lifestyle, cultural, psychological, and economic factors that might influence care or self-management
- Exercise history
- Symptoms related to complications
- Other cardiac risk factors, including smoking history
- Assessment for mood disorders
- Contraception and reproductive history
- Physical examination that includes eyes, mouth, thyroid, heart, abdomen, circulation (pulse), skin, breast exam, pelvic exam, and a neurological and foot exam
- Electrocardiogram
- Laboratory tests

Source: Adapted from the American Diabetes Association (Position Statement). Standards of Care for Patients with Diabetes. *Diabetes Care,* 29 (51) (2006).

➡ heart check-ups (EKGs or exercise tests, as recommended by your health care team)
➡ regular foot exams (in addition to routine foot care at home)
➡ dental check for gum disease every six months
➡ pre-pregnancy planning

There is nothing simple about good diabetes self-care, to be sure, but the benefits are well worth the effort.

To make it easier to track recommendations and know what to do and when, we've pulled everything together into one chart, Table 7.7. If you follow these guidelines, congratulations, you're on the pathway to healthier living.

Table 7.7 Medical care guidelines

Frequency	Goal	Lifestyle strategies	Medicines
Every medical visit			
Blood pressure check	130/80 mmHg	Salt restriction, weight loss, exercise, quit smoking	ACE inhibitors, ARBs, beta blockers, and/or diuretics
Weight measure	If loss necessary, 7–10 percent of original weight as initial goal		
Foot check	Check for sores, blisters, loss of sensation, other problems		
Review of glucose monitor log	Assess progress reaching target levels; change care plan if necessary		
Once per year			
Complete physical exam	Assess for physical and emotional problems; test and discuss progress reaching care goals and lifestyle changes; discuss birth control, fertility, or other applicable reproductive health issues		
Pap smear/pelvic exam	Part of annual exam		
Lipid tests (after 8-hour fast)			
—LDL	Less than 100 mg/dl	weight loss; exercise	Statins, niacin
—HDL	Raise above 50 mg/dl	weight loss; exercise	Niacin
—triglycerides	Less than 150 mg/dl	Get glucose under control; dietary changes, weight loss, exercise	Fibrates, statins
Comprehensive foot exam	More complete testing to identify high-risk feet with poor circulation and abnormal nerve function		
Kidney function test for urine microalbumin and a serum creatinine	To detect presence and progression of kidney disease	Glucose and blood pressure control; weight loss, less salt, increased exercise	ACE inhibitors, ARBs

Table 7.7   *(continued)*

Frequency	Goal	Lifestyle strategies	Medicines
Dilated eye examination	To detect presence and progression of diabetic eye disease (may be recommended more or less frequently)	Early detection, glucose and blood pressure control, laser therapy as needed	
Electrocardiogram	Annually after age 40		
Mammogram	Generally recommended annually at age 40 and above to detect signs of breast cancer		
Flu vaccination	To prevent that year's flus		
One-time Pneumococcal vaccine	Now recommended one time to prevent pneumonia and in some cases may have to be given again every ten years		
Two to four times a year HgbA$_{1c}$	Aim for less than 7 percent		
Two times a year Dental check-up	Check for presence of gum disease or other problems		

Once or twice a year
  Meet with diabetes nurse
    educator, after initial
    teaching of diabetes care			

8

Common
Questions and Resources

You will have many questions about this complex disease, since it affects every aspect of your daily life. In fact, if you don't have a lot of questions, you're probably not thinking enough about your diabetes. When you need help, you can always consult your health care team. You can also find a great deal of information in books, on the Internet, and from organizations such as the American Diabetes Association. Never before have there been so many resources to help you understand and cope with this disease.

We think of this book as a companion to help you get started on your journey with diabetes, letting you know what you as a woman can expect, and what it takes to provide basic diabetes care. As your companion, this book is here for you to refer to when a new issue arises.

This chapter covers some common questions that arise after diagnosis. We also point you to many other resources on diabetes. We firmly believe that knowledge, personal commitment, and the help of a good medical team are your best tools to master this disease.

HOW DO I GET ORGANIZED?

As you now know, managing diabetes is a lot of work. Like most women, you are probably juggling many responsibilities on top of controlling your diabetes. Somehow you must also find time to relax or take a walk for your physical and mental health. With so much on your mind, you can easily become forgetful or feel overwhelmed or stressed. Organization is the key to feeling in control.

ARRANGE YOUR MEDICAL CARE

The first step is to organize your medical care. You'll need to decide where you'll go and who will comprise your health care team. In most cases, you will need to find a doctor (either an endocrinologist or a primary care practitioner); a nurse or Certified Diabetes Educator (CDE); and a nutritionist. Many large hospitals and clinics have such teams already assembled in a Diabetes Center. If not, your primary care practitioner should be able to help you find the right health care experts for you. You'll want to be sure your providers have experience caring for people with diabetes and that they speak your language. If possible, try to arrange for medical care near your home. Once you've found a medical team, ask who is available in the event of an emergency.

ORGANIZE YOUR SUPPLIES

The second step is to organize your diabetes supplies. Find an accessible, central location to store everything related to your diabetes care. Organize a shelf or shelves so that you can easily see when you're running low on supplies or medications. (You should also note on a calendar when you will need refills.) Some supplies, like insulin and glucagon, are most stable when refrigerated. Others, like syringes, will need to be kept secure and out of the reach of children. A pill organizer will help you remember what medications you need to take and when.

It's also a good idea to keep extra supplies (including small bags of candy or juice to prevent or treat low blood sugar) on hand at work, in a bedside table, in your car, or in a travel bag you've set aside to take wherever you go. The rapidly acting carbohydrate should be readily available. Some people post a list of their medications and supplies on the refrigerator or a bulletin board for family members to refer to in case of an emergency.

ORGANIZE YOUR DAY

The third step is to manage your time. Most of us barely have enough time to get through the activities of daily living, let alone do all that's required for diabetes care. You may find it helpful to coordinate your testing schedule with some routine activities you do every day, such as brushing your teeth. Start by keeping a daily appointment book— alternatively, your team can supply you with a blood glucose "diary" or log—with plenty of space to write down everything you must do each day and at what time. You need a routine, so write down the time you take your medications and, if you take insulin, the dose; the time and results of your blood sugar monitoring; the time and duration of exercise; and of course the timing of meals and snacks. It often helps to mark down special events, such as parties or unusually intense exercise, that explain high or low blood glucose values. Keep track of medical appointments and note when you will need to refill supplies. In the beginning, adding more detail, such as meal composition and any deviations from your usual eating or exercise pattern, will help you understand fluctuations in blood sugar and make adjustments. Later on, when you understand better how your daily routine affects your diabetes and vice versa, you may not need to keep such a detailed record. Indicating your other responsibilities and "to-do" items may also help you stay organized. Check off each task as you accomplish it.

Here are some tips to help you organize your time and records:

➡ Get a daily appointment book with plenty of room to write down everything you must do each day and at what time. Keep track of glucose levels here or in a separate log.

➡ Mark down appointments and when to refill supplies.

➡ Indicate times to test glucose or take medicines. Use a timer or a watch alarm to remind you to check blood sugar levels or take medication at specific times.

➡ Schedule times to exercise regularly.

If you're technologically inclined, consider using a computer program or PDA (personal digital assistant) to help organize your life. PDAs are hand-held, computerized datebooks (also known as palm pilots) with software applications that can, for example, monitor your blood glucose readings, determine calories and nutrient content of foods, track your diet and exercise, and remind you to take your medications and keep your medical appointments.

One caution about these automated record-keepers is that they may be too automatic. Some people will dutifully store all their blood sugar results in their meters or hand-held devices and forget that they need to pay attention to their results every day in order to detect patterns and address them quickly.

Like all busy people, you need to prioritize. Sometimes you just have to say no and put diabetes first. Do the things that have to be done each day, and let some of the other household tasks or errands spill over to the next day. It's also a good idea to plan ahead as much as possible. Pack your snack for work the night before. Plan your meals, if not for the whole week ahead, then for the next day. If you plan and prioritize, you'll feel more in control of your life.

WHAT DO I DO WHEN I'M SICK?

Even a minor illness, like a cold or flu, can become a major problem if you don't stay on top of it. You need to plan ahead for when you're sick so that even if you don't have much energy, you'll know exactly what to do and already have the necessary supplies set aside.

When you are sick, your body is under stress. Stress can interfere with the effect of insulin and cause blood glucose levels to rise. Your appetite and food intake may change when you're ill, and this too may affect your blood sugar levels and medication needs. Whether you have type 1 or type 2 diabetes, you need to be alert to stop glucose levels from rising dangerously high or falling too low. That usually means monitoring your blood glucose levels more frequently than usual and checking your urine for ketones. Even if you can't keep food down, you will have to try to drink enough to stay hydrated and gradually try to eat foods from a sick-day food plan that you work out in advance with your physician or diabetes educator.

The sick-day plan will include information on how often to monitor blood glucose, when to test for ketones (for example, when your glucose is over 300 mg/dl or when you have gastrointestinal symptoms like nausea or vomiting), what medicines to take, which foods you should try to eat, and when you should call someone on your health care team. If you are unable to take your oral medicines during an illness, you might have to take insulin temporarily, even if you don't usually.

Although you may need to change your insulin doses when you are ill, if you have type 1 diabetes you should *never* stop taking your insulin during an illness. If you have type 2 diabetes and are treated with insulin, you may need to adjust or even stop your insulin during an illness, but you need to talk to your team first. When in doubt, call or page your health care team to discuss what to do with your medications. Don't wait.

You should also be aware that some over-the-counter cold medicines can affect blood sugar: decongestants can raise glucose levels, and some cough syrups contain sugar, so check the ingredients and ask the pharmacist if you are not sure which over-the-counter remedies are safe for you.

SICK-DAY PLANS

- Check your blood glucose levels more frequently than usual, for example, every four hours.

- Keep taking your insulin and diabetes pills. Even if you can't keep food down, you still need your medication, though you may require a lower dose. Check with your medical provider.

- Drink at least a cup of water every hour you're awake.

- If you can't eat your usual food, drink juice or eat crackers, popsicles, or soup.

- If you can't eat at all, drink clear liquids such as ginger ale.

- If you have type 1 diabetes, test your urine for ketones if

    –your blood glucose is over 300; or if

    –you can't keep food or liquids down.

- Call your health care provider right away if you have any of the following problems:

    –your blood glucose has been over 300 for longer than one day;

    –you have moderate to large amounts of ketones in your urine;

    –you feel sleepier than usual;

    –you have trouble breathing;

    –you can't think clearly;

    –you throw up more than once or can't take liquids because of nausea or vomiting;

    –you've had diarrhea for more than six hours;

    –you have chest pain.

Source: Adapted from "Taking Care of Your Diabetes at Special Times," National Diabetes Information Clearinghouse (http://diabetes.niddk.nih.gov/dm/pubs/type1and2/specialtimes.htm#1).

It is critical that you remain well hydrated and drink lots of fluids when you are ill. If you are unable to keep food down, your team may advise you to have liquids with sugar in them, such as fruit juices or nondiet ginger ale. If you're sick enough to require this type of attention, make sure that you call your health care providers for advice. If you can't even keep fluids down—for example, if you have a gastroin-

WHAT IS CONSIDERED AN EMERGENCY SITUATION?

Very low or very high blood sugar readings can be emergency situations. Low blood sugars can result if you take too much medication (insulin or sulfonylureas), miss a meal, get more exercise than usual, or drink too much alcohol. High blood sugars can occur when you take too little medication, eat more than usual (especially carbohydrates), or when you are ill.

Call your medical provider if your blood glucose reading is less than 70 mg/dl and cannot be explained, or more than 300 mg/dl, and if:

- you have more than two high readings in a row and cannot explain why your sugars are high;
- you have associated symptoms of diabetes (excessive thirst, hunger, urination, fatigue, weight loss);
- you have type 1 diabetes and moderate or large amounts of ketones in your urine; or
- you are sick.

The symptoms of low blood sugar may be:

- nervousness
- trembling
- sweating
- fast heart rate
- clamminess
- irritability
- confusion
- sleepiness
- weakness
- hunger
- dizziness
- double vision
- if severe, loss of consciousness, seizures, coma

For any low blood sugar, you should do the following:

1. Test your blood glucose, if possible.
2. If you can't test, treat yourself as below. It's better to be safe than sorry.

3. If your reading is less than 70 mg/dl, then eat or drink:
- 2–5 glucose tablets;
- 2 teaspoons of sugar or honey;
- 1 cup milk;
- 1/2 cup of juice or soda (not diet); or
- 5–7 Lifesaver candies.

4. Retest your blood sugar in 15 minutes; if it's still low, repeat step 3.

---

testinal "bug" or flu—you may need to go to an emergency room or hospital to be given intravenous fluids. The sooner you get help, the sooner you'll feel better. Remember, when in doubt, call your health care providers.

There is no way yet to prevent the common cold, but you can reduce your risk of getting viral influenza (the "flu") with an annual flu shot. Although not 100 percent effective, the vaccine improves your chances of getting through the winter months without the flu and is highly recommended for people with diabetes. You should also get a pneumonia shot (a vaccine against the most common forms of bacterial pneumonia), since a bout of pneumonia will complicate your diabetes. You only need the shot once, with a booster every five to ten years.

HOW SHOULD I PREPARE FOR TRAVEL?

Preparation is also key before traveling, particularly if you are flying. In the wake of the September 11 terrorist hijackings, there are very strict security regulations for how passengers may carry diabetes supplies onto airplanes. Air travel these days takes a lot of patience, good humor, and extra snacks. Delays, unpredictability, and changing time zones go with the territory.

Here are some tips for travel near or far:

➡ Keep a travel bag with you that has all your diabetes supplies: more than enough oral medications or insulin to cover the days of your trip, a glucose meter (and extra batteries), capped lancets, other medications you might need (antidiarrhea or antinausea drugs, for example).

➡ Bring plenty of snacks—crackers, fruit, pretzels, and juice—for the long lines and delays.

➡ If you are crossing several time zones, have someone on your health care team help you figure out the timing of your insulin injections and other medications and meals.

➡ Wear comfortable shoes and don't walk barefoot.

➡ Always carry or wear a medical bracelet or necklace that identifies you as having diabetes, in case of emergency.

➡ Bring a letter from your physician listing all the diabetes supplies you use, any allergies or food restrictions, and contact information for emergencies; bring prescriptions for medications you take in case they are lost.

➡ If you take insulin, carry your syringes with you on the plane; your physician should include this information in your "travel letter."

➡ If you use insulin, protect it from extremes of temperature (keep it cool, if possible, but *not* frozen).

➡ Remember that X-ray equipment won't hurt your diabetes devices or medicines.

➡ However you are traveling, try to take breaks and walk around a bit to stretch your legs.

➡ Check your blood sugars more frequently when traveling to prevent hypoglycemia. Check your blood sugar before you start driving and at regular intervals.

Flying within the United States: It is important to realize that what to you is medical treatment is to a security person a potential threat. Syringes and lancing devices will be perceived as dangerous weapons unless you can prove they are for your diabetes care. In the past, a letter from your physician documenting your need was sufficient, but because it is possible to forge such documents, you now must bring all your medicines and supplies in original pharmacy packages with prescription labels. Lancets must be capped and you must

Various kinds of medical identification

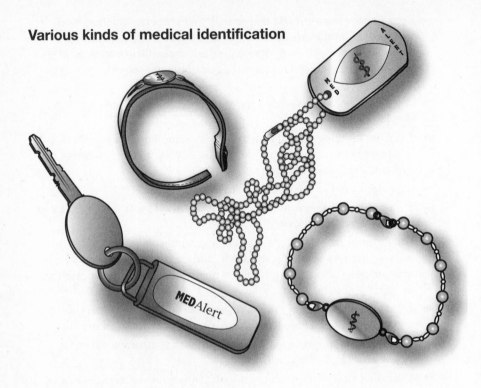

Several types of medical IDs are available. Pick one that works for you.

prove that you use them for glucose monitoring by showing your meter with its brand name printed on it. You must also show that the brand name matches the brand on your test strips. A security officer may even ask to check through your food. Be cooperative, but if you feel harassed, then ask to speak with the security manager or a "complaint resolution officer."

Not all domestic flights offer meals anymore. Call ahead and ask. Order a diabetic meal if they have one or, if not, bring your own meal on board. Ask if an attendant can heat it up for you, if necessary.

Flying outside the United States: To avoid any surprises, contact the foreign embassy of any country you are visiting to see if they have regulations governing travel with diabetes supplies. Many foreign countries have embassies in Washington, D.C.; information on how to

CHECKLIST FOR TRAVELING WITH INSULIN

Be sure to pack:

• Twice the amount of insulin, syringes, insulin pen, and cartridges you will need

• Glucose meter. Put in new batteries before you go. Take a spare meter if you have one.

• Test strips

• Extra batteries for meter

• Lancing device and lancets

• Ketone test strips

• Glucagon

• Glucose tabs or gel, Lifesavers, or other carbohydrates to treat lows

• Medical identification. Wear it!

• Prescriptions for insulin, syringes, and other medications

• Doctor's letter

• Water—one or two 16-ounce bottles

• Meal equivalent—sandwich, fruit, cookie, vegetables. Check with your airline or travel agent to see if there are any restrictions on boarding with fruits and vegetables.

• Snacks—granola bars, pretzels, mini bagels, string cheese, crackers, fruit

• Alcohol pads or other cleansing agent

• Tissues

• Fanny pack or backpack

• Two pairs of comfortable, well-made walking shoes

• First-aid supplies—adhesive bandages, gauze, ace bandages, antibiotic ointment, etc.

• Sharps container

• Antinausea and antidiarrhea pills

• Cold pack

• Pain medication—aspirin, acetaminophen, ibuprofen

• Insect repellent, sunscreen, and sunglasses

Pump users should also carry:

• Extra batteries

• Extra infusion sets, cartridges, and occlusive dressings

- IV Prep or other antibacterial cleanser
- Antibiotic ointment
- Alternate basal insulin and syringes—Lantus or NPH—especially if you do not have a back-up pump
- Extra pump. Check with the manufacturer, as many will provide a loaner for international travel.

Source: Adapted from Terry Lumber and Patricia Strainic, "Have Insulin, Will Travel: Planning Ahead Will Make Traveling with Insulin Smooth Sailing," *Diabetes Forecast* (August 2005), pp. 51–54.

---

contact them can be found online at embassy.org. You should also learn how to say such phrases as "I have diabetes" or "sugar or orange juice, please," in languages of the countries you'll be visiting.

IS IT SAFE TO DRIVE A CAR?

With a few exceptions, there is no reason that someone with diabetes cannot safely drive a car. If you are treated with insulin or a sulfonylurea, becoming hypoglycemic while driving is the main risk. If you don't recognize and deal with hypoglycemia in a timely fashion, it can lead to moving violations (speeding, running a red light, for example) or accidents. An international study published in *Diabetes Care* in August 2003 found that drivers with type 1 diabetes are at increased risk for driving mishaps, but type 2 diabetic drivers, even those on insulin, appear not to be. (This statistical conclusion does not, however, mean that women with type 2 diabetes treated with insulin are not at risk for having severe, potentially dangerous hypoglycemia.) Those with type 1 diabetes who were found to be particularly prone to car accidents were those who monitored their blood glucose less frequently and those who injected their insulin as opposed to using a pump. (This also does not mean that pump therapy safeguards you from hypoglycemia.)

You can take the following precautions to ensure driving safety, particularly when traveling long distances:

➡ Do not drive if your blood glucose level is too low. If you take insulin and your level is less than 100 mg/dl or if your blood glucose is likely to fall—after exercise, for example—have a carbohydrate snack. It's always better to be safe than sorry.

➡ Keep fast-acting sugar snacks and your glucose meter within easy reach at all times.

➡ Pull over to the side of the road as soon as you feel any symptoms of hypoglycemia: sleepiness, dizziness, or confusion; or if you have blurred vision. Check your blood sugar and treat yourself. Even if you can't test your blood sugar, treat yourself. When in doubt, respond as if you're hypoglycemic. Wait to drive again until you have fully recovered.

➡ Keep to regular meal times; take frequent breaks from driving.

Whether you have type 1 or type 2 diabetes, it is a good idea to discuss driving with someone on your health care team. Some complications resulting from diabetes—eye problems, leg numbness, hypoglycemic unawareness—may mean you need special adaptations to drive or that you shouldn't drive at all.

There are extra reasons that anyone with diabetes shouldn't drive after drinking alcohol, even small amounts. Alcohol may lower blood glucose and can increase the risk of severe hypoglycemia. The hypoglycemia may even occur several hours after drinking, when the effects of the alcohol have worn off. The symptoms can be confused with drunkenness, and if that happens, you may not get the treatment you need.

SHOULD I TELL MY EMPLOYER I HAVE DIABETES?

Women today make up close to 50 percent of the workforce, and 99 out of every 100 women will work for pay at some point in their lives, according to the U.S. Department of Labor's Women's Bureau. Whether you are home or at work, diabetes affects your life, and your life affects your diabetes. Wherever you are, you have to try to maintain your monitoring, medication, and eating routines. Many women wonder whether they should tell co-workers or supervisors that they have diabetes, and what to do if they feel they've been discriminated against, either because they have diabetes or because they are overweight or obese.

Generally speaking, although everyone is entitled to her privacy, there is no reason to hide the fact that you have diabetes. It's merely another piece of information about your life, and one that may be important to help those around you provide support and assistance, if you should need it. If you are treated with insulin, let trusted people around you know, in case you have hypoglycemia and need assistance. Sometimes, hypoglycemia can sneak up on you, especially if you suffer from "hypoglycemia unawareness," and your co-workers may notice the signs before you do. If they know you have diabetes, they will be in a better position to get you a snack or help out in other ways. Women who work in jobs that may be hazardous, such as operating heavy equipment or machinery, must be especially careful since an episode of hypoglycemia could lead to serious injury to themselves or others.

On the other hand, it is also understandable if you consider your health issues to be your private business. But don't let that stop you from taking steps to maintain your care routine at work, for example, by requesting a lunch break at the same time every day. You can always tell your supervisor that you're following doctor's orders without specifying why, and if necessary you can provide a note from your physician to that effect.

In the past, employers sometimes discriminated against people with diabetes—didn't hire them or treat them fairly on the job—solely because of the disease. The Americans with Disabilities Act (ADA), passed in 1990, was designed to prevent such discrimination. Even if you are not "disabled" according to the criteria of the law, the ADA protects you if an employer discriminates against you because he or she thinks or acts as if diabetes is an impairment. You cannot be discriminated against as long as you are qualified for the job and can perform the duties required of your position.

According to the law, you are disabled if:

→ You have a physical or mental impairment that greatly limits one or more major life activities (such as seeing, hearing, walking, caring for oneself, and working).

→ You once had such an impairment.

→ Others regard you as having such an impairment.

Less well protected legally are those who are discriminated against for being overweight. A 1999 review conducted at Western Michigan University of twenty-nine research studies found evidence of discrimination against overweight people at every stage of employment from hiring practices, salaries, job placement and promotion, to discipline and firings. Studies have found that women in particular may be discriminated against on the basis of weight. Two studies, for example, reported that the wages of mildly obese white women were 5.9 percent lower than those of normal-weight white women for comparable jobs, and those of morbidly obese women were 24.1 percent lower (American Obesity Association: www.obesity.org/discrimination/employment.shtml). There is also some evidence that the job performance of overweight women is evaluated more negatively than that of overweight men.

The ADA does not specifically include obesity as a disability. But an increasing number of court cases have supported morbid obesity as a disability, qualifying plaintiffs for ADA protection. That is not the case for those who are overweight or less obese (the majority of workers!), however. The American Obesity Association works to protect the rights of those who are obese and can provide a great deal of legal, health, and practical information (see the resource list at the end of this chapter).

HOW CAN I EAT OUT WITHOUT BLOWING MY DIET?

Eating out is a treat, but it doesn't have to be a reason to overindulge or go off your meal plan. Whether you are out to eat at a friend's, a local restaurant, a party, or a fast-food place, you can eat healthfully and not sacrifice a good time.

Recognizing that eating out is one of the top reasons that people go off their diets, the Diabetes Prevention Program included counseling on "four keys to healthy eating out":

→ *Plan ahead.* Pick a restaurant that has low-fat or heart-healthy choices. Try to limit your daily fat grams for the rest of the day so you can use them when you're out. Know what you want to order so you're not tempted by excessively high calorie, high-fat items on the menu. If you're invited to someone's house, let your host know ahead of time about your dietary restrictions. Eat a little snack before you go out.

→ *Ask for what you want.* Restaurants stay in business by giving you, the customer, what you want. Be friendly about it, but don't hesitate to ask for special preparations: sauce on the side, for example, or a broiled entrée instead of a fried one. Ask about the size of portions, and if they're too big, see if they can prepare the dish in an appetizer size, share an entrée with a friend, or ask the waiter to put half in a "doggie bag" *before* serving it to you.

→ *Take charge of what's around you.* Be the first to order and you won't be tempted by what the others are ordering. If you're at a buffet party, look at all the food being offered before carefully selecting a few favorites to fill one small plate; then don't go back. Be ready with a confident answer to those who may try to encourage you to eat something you shouldn't.

→ *Choose foods carefully.* Know your restrictions—low salt, a certain number of carbohydrate or fat grams, or low cholesterol—and choose accordingly. Have fruit or sherbet for dessert, or share a dessert with a friend (accounting for its calories, fat grams, and carbs, of course).

It's helpful to think of the kinds of problems you've encountered in the past when eating out. What were you tempted by, what led you astray? Plan ahead and think about what you can say or do to avoid slipping the next time.

HOW CAN I QUIT SMOKING?

Please do not skip this section if you are among the 25 percent or so of Americans who smoke cigarettes. Smoking can have devastating health consequences for all women, but particularly for women with either type 1 or type 2 diabetes, as they are already at increased risk for cardiovascular disease. Smoking is also related to the development of nephropathy, neuropathy, and possibly retinopathy.

Nicotine is a powerful addiction but it can be beaten. The incentives are your own health, the health of children you may have now or in the future, and the health of anyone around you who might breathe in your second-hand smoke. It may take several tries to quit, but support is available to help you succeed.

Talk to someone on your health care team about quitting. They can refer you to a local program to support you in your efforts. There is good evidence that those who try to quit by enrolling in a support program are more likely to succeed than those who try on their own. Your health care team can also prescribe one of the therapies available to lessen the urge to smoke. These include nicotine gum, a patch, an inhaler, oral medications such as bupropion (Zyban), or a nasal spray. They can also adapt your diabetes care plan to minimize the weight gain that often occurs after quitting. Weight gain should not be a reason not to quit, though you should anticipate the possibility by building more exercise into your day. You'll need to be extra vigilant not to respond to the craving for tobacco by eating fattening foods.

One suggestion: if you have a craving for a cigarette, distract yourself for the five minutes it takes for the craving to pass. Chew sugarless gum, eat nonbuttered popcorn, or keep your hands busy by knitting, doing a crossword puzzle, or engaging in some sort of physical activity.

The first step to quitting is to set a date. Don't pick a time when you're already stressed out, or around a holiday, when there's extra food around. But plan the date enough in advance that you can prepare ways to handle cravings and strategies to break old patterns. For example, have your morning coffee in a different location or drink tea instead, anything to change the coffee-and-a-cigarette routine. Have activities lined up to keep you busy. And be ready to toss out ashtrays and everything that reminds you of cigarettes. Add up all the money you'll save.

ARE THERE SOLUTIONS FOR EXTREME OBESITY?

Obesity can significantly shorten life. Numerous studies have shown the short-term health benefits of decreasing weight. The few studies that have looked at longer-term weight loss have shown it has major benefits. The lifestyle changes in diet and activity described in this book are key to healthy weight loss for women of every size. But clearly if you have 100 or more pounds to lose, you are faced with a formidable task. Particularly if you are already experiencing diabetes and other health problems, the benefits of such measures as bariatric surgery for obesity may well exceed the risks.

The first approach will always be to lose weight through dietary changes and increased activity. The typical goal is to lose a pound every week or ten days by reducing your usual intake of calories by 400 to 500 per day. Increasing caloric expenditure will also help adjust your energy balance to promote weight loss. Although dramatic weight loss may be achieved in the short term with more radical dietary approaches such as "very low calorie" diets, in which calories are limited to less than 800 per day, or the use of liquid meal replacements, these strategies are generally not recommended because their long-term success is very limited. If you decide to try a more radical diet, you will need to be closely monitored by your health care team. Behavior therapy, active monitoring of your progress through food diaries, follow-up from your health care team, and exercise are all ingredients to successful long-term weight loss.

Drugs that promote weight loss are available, but they are all relatively ineffective, leading to only small weight loss. Drugs should never be used instead of lifestyle efforts but should complement them. The three weight-loss medications currently approved for long-term use are fenfluramine (Pondimin), sibutramine (Meridia), and orlistat (Xenical). Fenfluramine, the oldest of the prescription drugs currently available, suppresses appetite. Sibutramine, another appetite suppressant, can increase blood pressure and heart rate, and may not be appropriate for those with high blood pressure or heart disease. Orlistat keeps about one-third of the fat eaten from being absorbed by the body; the result is weight loss, lowered blood glucose, and improved cholesterol levels. Further studies need to be done on the safety of using these drugs beyond two years. We do know, however, that weight is often regained after the drugs are discontinued.

The most drastic—and effective—solution to extreme obesity is bariatric surgery, in which the size of the stomach is reduced and, in some procedures, part of the small intestine is bypassed. Surgery, such as gastric bypass, produces rapid and, more important, sustained weight loss and improves insulin and glucose levels. Weight loss of about 60 percent of excess weight, with an average of 75 to 100 pounds, is typical during the first year. Glucose levels improve right after surgery, in fact even before much weight is lost.

There are serious risks involved with these surgeries, however. Estimates vary, but death after bariatric surgery occurs in one of every one hundred to two hundred cases. Part of the risk is secondary to complications that can occur in very obese people with any kind of anesthesia and surgery, such as respiratory problems, blood clots in the legs or lungs, or heart attacks.

In the most common procedure, the gastric bypass, the stomach is reduced to a small pouch and stapled shut. The small stomach pouch is attached at a point farther down on the small intestine, effectively "bypassing" part of the small intestine where calories and vitamins are absorbed. The most common complications specific to this surgery are for a staple or suture to break, allowing the stomach's contents to leak into other parts of the body, or for the connection between the stomach pouch and the intestine to leak. These problems can cause an infection that can be fatal. If you're considering bariatric surgery, it is extremely important to find an experienced surgeon and to consider carefully if this is the right approach for you.

A somewhat newer procedure, which can be performed endoscopically without a major incision, is gastric "banding." In this surgery, a small inflatable donut is placed around the stomach. When it is inflated, it creates a small gastric pouch as with surgical stapling; however, the band is not permanent and can be removed or adjusted. Weight loss is not as great with banding as with the stapling and bypass procedure, but the risks are probably lower.

CAN I SAFELY HAVE A BABY?

It is very common for women to wonder if diabetes will affect their ability to get pregnant. They want to make sure pregnancy is safe for them and their baby. And they worry if their future children will get diabetes.

We cover each of these issues in greater detail in Chapter 5. But to summarize: these days a woman with diabetes who keeps her blood glucose levels near normal both before and during pregnancy has almost the same chance of delivering a healthy baby as a woman without diabetes. It is critical, however, to involve your health care team in preparing for pregnancy many months before you stop using contraceptives. Otherwise, you have a greater risk of miscarriage or fetal malformations.

Some of your diabetic complications, such as retinopathy, nephropathy, and neuropathy, may worsen during pregnancy, but they often return to the prepregnancy state after delivery. Pregnancy does not appear to increase the risk of developing these complications permanently.

Women with type 2 diabetes and PCOS may have trouble getting pregnant, but this can often be remedied through treatment of PCOS.

Women with type 1 whose diabetes is well controlled are not much more likely to have fertility problems than women without diabetes.

It is less clear, however, how to know whether your baby is likely to get diabetes. Both type 1 and type 2 diabetes can be inherited. Having a first-degree relative (parent or sibling) with diabetes increases a child's chances of getting the same type of the disease. But many children and adults get diabetes when no one else in their families has it. There are many variables underlying inheritance and development of diabetes that are not well understood. This is usually not a reason to avoid pregnancy.

DOES MENOPAUSE CAUSE OR WORSEN DIABETES?

Menopause does not cause diabetes, though you may coincidently have been diagnosed with diabetes at the same time you entered menopause. Nor does menopause worsen diabetes. The fluctuating hormones that characterize perimenopause and menopause, however, can make controlling blood glucose levels more challenging. The hormonal changes in concert with erratic blood glucose levels can intensify the mood swings, fatigue, and hot flashes that can occur around the time of menopause. It can certainly feel as if your diabetes is worse at this time of life.

As described in Chapter 5, menopause does make women, and especially women with diabetes, more prone to certain medical problems. Yeast infections and urinary tract infections are more likely at this time, for example. So is weight gain. And with the reduction of estrogen, lipid profiles change in a way that is even less heart-protective. Already at high risk for cardiovascular problems, women with diabetes are at even greater risk at menopause.

Diabetes doesn't worsen at menopause. But if you have diabetes, menopause is a good time to have your care plan reassessed. You may need new medications or a change in your diet and activity level.

DO OLDER WOMEN WITH DIABETES NEED SPECIAL CARE?

About one out of every five women over age sixty-five has diabetes. Many older women with the disease stay active and highly motivated to take care of themselves. For them the goals of diabetes care are the same as they are for women of all ages.

But the challenges of living with diabetes can become daunting for women in their older years. Many are confronted not only with managing diabetes but with other impairments as well, such as arthritis, reduced vision, heart disease, and memory loss. Older women are at greater risk of depression, urinary incontinence, falls, and chronic pain. Women over age sixty-five are more than twice as likely as men of the same age to live in poverty.

If you have arthritis or have had a stroke, it may be physically difficult for you to operate your blood glucose monitor. If you have vision problems, you may not be able to inspect your feet properly or read the dosage markings on a syringe. The memory loss that can be associated with diabetes, aging, and cardiovascular disease makes under-medication or over-medication more likely. Multiple health issues make it difficult to stay motivated to take care of yourself and eat properly. In addition to your diabetes medications, you are likely to be treated with several blood pressure medicines, a cholesterol-lowering medicine, an aspirin, and other medications to treat ailments that become increasingly common with older age. You may find yourself frail, less mobile, and living alone. Money may be an issue.

Although sometimes treatment goals need to be modified, accommodations can often be made in the care plan for older people. Self-care devices are available for those with reduced vision. Age, obesity, and other health problems may limit exercise, but your health care team can help you find alternative activities that are realistic and safe. You can make changes to your meal plan if certain foods cause digestive problems. If arthritis and vision problems make mixing insulin difficult, you can try insulin pens with premixed insulin. There are many ways to equip your home to prevent falls.

Family involvement and social supports become more critical than ever in the older years. Your health care team can adapt your diabetes care plan on the basis of your changing needs and the realities of your lifestyle, and they can help you locate any social services you need to meet the goals for care. As in each phase of life, the older years bring new challenges that can be met with dignity.

HOW DO I FIND HEALTH CARE THAT RESPECTS MY CULTURE?

Recognizing that more than ever before the United States is a melting pot of diverse groups, health care institutions are struggling to ensure that the care they deliver is "culturally competent." At a basic level this comes down to trying to treat a disease in the context of a patient's culture—beliefs, customs, and habits that affect her understanding of her illness and what she has to do to treat it. This respect for different cultures and lifestyles is particularly important in the care of diabetes, which is so dependent on lifestyle changes. Moreover, diabetes is more common among minorities, including Latino/Hispanic Americans, African Americans, Asian Americans, and Native Americans.

Culturally competent care is more than handing someone a pamphlet on diabetes written in Spanish or Chinese. It means having a professional translator available if one is necessary and not relying on a family member to translate. It also means that the health care provider asks open-ended questions to understand an individual's perspective on her disease. What do you think caused it? Are there traditional ways of treating diabetes in your culture? What are the specific behaviors that led to your being overweight, and what barriers are there to effective diabetes therapy?

Although diabetes educators of the same cultural background as the patients can be enormously helpful, health care providers from different backgrounds can also be effective if they take the time to understand their patients' beliefs and lifestyles and adapt recommendations for healthy changes that are culturally appropriate.

The federal government has set standards for reducing the health disparities in care for ethnic and racial minorities in the United States. The result is a much greater understanding in hospitals and general medical practices around the country that mere competence at care is not enough. When an individual's cultural orientation is part of the equation, the outcome will be a lot better in terms of mutual respect, adherence to treatment plans, and prevention of complications.

If you feel you are not getting this kind of respect, speak with a patient advocate at the clinic or hospital where you receive services. Community-based service organizations can also sometimes guide or direct you to local care that is more culturally attuned to your needs.

DO ALTERNATIVE TREATMENTS HELP?

An increasing number of Americans, including those with diabetes, are turning to a wide variety of alternative medicines and practices. Some of the approaches that have been studied as a complement to diabetes care include acupuncture (for relief from the pain of neuropathy), massage therapy, biofeedback, relaxation techniques, and yoga. Various herbs and vitamin and mineral supplements are also purported to help lower blood glucose.

In Western medicine these approaches are termed "alternative" or "complementary" treatments. Many of them have not yet been proven effective through controlled clinical trials involving large numbers of people, the basis of sound scientific method. Western scientists are skeptical of alternative treatments because many supposed wonder drugs have turned out not to work after being tested in clinical trials. Some herbal remedies might help manage diabetes, but we don't yet have enough evidence on most of them to know. Until we do, the main thing you need to determine before you try an alternative medication is if it is safe and without side effects. It is also important to let your health care provider know if you plan to try one or are currently taking one. Some herbal preparations do not interact well with traditional medicines. Examples include garlic and fenugreek, herbs that may increase the blood-thinning effect of warfarin, taken to prevent blood clots.

Just because most of these herbs are natural and derived from plants does not automatically make them safe or better than more traditional Western medications. On the other hand, the unproven herb of today may be an approved medicine of tomorrow. Metformin, for example, is derived from the flowering plant *Galega officinalis.* Just know that if you are taking something that is as yet unproven, you are an experimental guinea pig. Herbal products in this country are not regulated by the FDA as drugs are. They do not go through the rigorous approval process to prove safety and effectiveness that the FDA requires for prescription drugs. Also, the manufacturing and packaging of these products is not well regulated, so one bottle may be very different from another.

The best advice is to get solid information before trying an herb or other supplement. One good source is a paper published in April 2003 in the medical journal *Diabetes Care* (volume 26, number 4), written by Harvard Medical School physicians in the Division for Research and Education in Complementary and Integrative Medical Therapies. They reviewed all the published literature on herbs and supplements for diabetes control and concluded that there was not enough evidence to prove the effectiveness of any of them, although they appeared generally safe. The best positive evidence they found was for *Coccinia indica* (an herb used in the East Indian healing system Ayurveda) and American ginseng. They cited other herbs that might also be promising but needed more research, such as *Aloe vera* and *Gymnema sylvestre* (another Ayurvedic herb). We review some of the current evidence in Appendix 9.

The National Center for Complementary and Alternative Medicine, which is part of the National Institutes of Health, also uses scientific methods to evaluate herbal and other alternative methods of treatment.

HOW WILL I PAY FOR ALL
THE SUPPLIES I NEED?

If you have diabetes, the best situation is to be enrolled in a group health plan through your employer or your spouse's employer. Usually such plans cover the costs of medical care, diabetes education, and supplies (glucose meter, test strips, lancets, and so on). However, the amount of coverage varies from policy to policy.

States have different regulations for what must be covered. For example, forty-six states (excluding Alabama, Idaho, Ohio, and North Dakota) require carriers to cover diabetes education, equipment, and supplies. By federal law, Medicare covers most of the costs of glucose meters, strips, lancets, self-management training, and diabetes screening tests for those considered at high risk. Medicaid (for those with low income who are eligible) will reimburse patients for most diabetes medications, although coverage varies from state to state.

Problems can arise when you try to switch insurers or, if underinsured or uninsured, you try to enroll in a new group plan or get individual insurance. Often insurers have a period of time during which they are not obligated to pay for treatments related to a medical condition you already had. In most states, individual insurers can decide not to cover you if you have a pre-existing condition (something that employee-sponsored group plans cannot do). Roughly thirty states offer "high-risk pools" for those who have been turned down by insurers, though this kind of coverage is expensive.

It can be very confusing trying to understand the various insurance options to which you might be entitled. The Georgetown University Health Policy Institute has written consumer guides for each state on how to get and keep health insurance on the basis of state regulations. These guides—which also include consumer protections when buying group or individual insurance, limitations for pre-existing conditions, and financial assistance—are available online at www.healthinsuranceinfo.net. The American Diabetes Association also provides information on health insurance for people with diabetes, as does the National Institute of Diabetes and Kidney Disease's National Diabetes Information Clearinghouse (see contact information at the end of this chapter).

Even with insurance, you will still have to cover out-of-pocket costs for medications, such as co-pays. Some people with diabetes cut back on their prescribed medications for financial reasons. This is strongly discouraged. If you are having trouble paying for your medications, talk to someone on your health care team. He or she may be able to prescribe less costly generic drug alternatives, give you free samples, or point you to assistance programs.

Test strips for glucose monitors are sometimes not adequately covered in insurance plans, but their costs can vary significantly from one pharmacy to another. It pays to shop around. And don't forget to consider the cost of test strips when comparing glucose monitors before purchasing one.

SHOULD I JOIN A CLINICAL TRIAL?

At some time, you may hear about an option to join a clinical trial, a research study that uses humans as subjects to answer specific medical questions, such as, is a new oral medication better than the ones currently being used? Or perhaps you are interested in finding out if there are any trials of new treatments for a complication of diabetes you are experiencing. Before signing on to a study, you need to do your homework.

Clinical trials are the primary way we develop and evaluate potential new treatments. Many of the advances in the care and prevention of diabetes and its complications have been made through clinical trials. We described several of the largest trials in Chapter 3. The Diabetes Prevention Program study, for example, told us that type 2 diabetes can be prevented or at least delayed through a 5 to 10 percent reduction in body weight and at least thirty minutes of physical activity each day. The results were so dramatic in the group that followed these lifestyle modifications that the trial was stopped one year earlier than planned so that the results could be reported and everybody at risk for diabetes could benefit. You should know, however, that results are not always this dramatic, and sometimes people in the group trying new medications experience unpleasant side effects. In short, the new treatment being studied may or may not benefit you personally. But learning that something doesn't work is also important in the ongoing quest to find better agents and treatments for diabetes and its complications.

Before joining a clinical trial, you should understand what is being tested and how, the risks and benefits, the commitment required of you (extra office visits and tests, for example), and how patient safety is being ensured. You should usually discuss joining a clinical trial with your health care team, who can determine whether it will interfere with your current therapy. You will be required to sign an "informed consent" form, signifying that you understand all the key facts about the study and agree to participate. The form does not bind you to the study, though the investigators hope you will complete it; you can always opt out at any time. And even if you are enrolled in a clinical trial, you will usually continue your normal care routine with your diabetes health care team.

Several key websites can provide information on clinical trials that are enrolling participants in your area. The National Institutes of Health has a comprehensive site at www.clinicaltrials.gov. In addition to listing federal and privately funded trials, it has general information on clinical trials and links to other consumer health sources. You can also consult www.centerwatch.com for information on more than 41,000 industry- and government-supported clinical trials. Internet access is usually offered free of charge at local public libraries.

RESOURCES

Thousands of books, pamphlets, magazines, and websites provide information about diabetes. The list below is just a sampling, mostly including what is available free of charge through the Internet. If you don't have Internet access at home, check your local public library. Any of these organizations can also be contacted by phone or mail.

The websites listed below are affiliated with the government and professional associations and are reliable. Most hospitals and medical centers also have printed and electronic information on diabetes.

USEFUL WEBSITES

www.aadi.joslin.harvard.edu (Asian American Diabetes Initiative)

www.bsc.gwu.edu/dpp/index.htmlvdoc (Diabetes Prevention Program)

www.cdc.gov/diabetes (Center for Disease Control and Prevention's diabetes division)

www.childrenwithdiabetes.com

www.diabetes.org (American Diabetes Association)

www.diabetesnet.com

www.diabetesnews.com

www.diabetes.niddk.nih.gov (National Diabetes Information Clearinghouse)

www.diabetes123.com

www.ediet.com

www.ethnomed.org (information in different languages)

www.healthinsuranceinfo.net (Georgetown University Health Policy Institute)

www.insulin-pumpers.org

www.jdrf.org (Juvenile Diabetes Research Foundation)

www.joslin.org (Joslin Diabetes Center)

www.metrokc.gov/health/reach/diabetes.htm

www.ndep.nih.gov (National Diabetes Education Program)

www.nlm.nih.gov/medlineplus/diabetes.html (National Library of Medicine)

www.spiral.tufts.edu (information in multiple languages)

There is plenty of information and support out there when you're ready for it. The power is within you to make the changes necessary to prevent or gain control of this disease. Now it is up to you.

American Association of Diabetes Educators (AADE): The professional society for diabetes educators. Its website features a public section with general information on diabetes, diabetes educators, and links to companies producing diabetes products, among other helpful links.

> AADE
> 100 W. Monroe, Suite 400
> Chicago, IL 60603
> 1-800-338-3633
> www.aadenet.org

American Diabetes Association: An organization that publishes books and magazines, advocates for the rights of those with diabetes, sponsors community events, and maintains a comprehensive website with diabetes information for consumers and health care professionals. The ADA publishes three medical journals—*Diabetes, Diabetes Care,* and *Diabetes Spectrum*—and a consumer magazine, *Diabetes Forecast,* which features an annual Resource Guide on new diabetes products and medications every January (www.diabetes.org/diabetes-forecast/resource-guide.jsp).

> American Diabetes Association
> 1701 North Beauregard St.
> Alexandria, VA 22311
> 1-800-342-2383
> www.diabetes.org
> email: askada@diabetes.org (ask diabetes-related questions or request a
> diabetes information packet)

American Dietetic Association: An organization that provides nutrition information; maintains a searchable database of registered dietitians; and publishes (for a fee) diabetes education materials, including meal plans using various ethnic and regional foods.

> American Dietetic Association (headquarters)
> 120 South Riverside Plaza, Suite 2000
> Chicago, IL 60606-6995
> 1-800-877-1600
> www.eatright.org

American Heart Association: A national organization that provides information on the warning signs and prevention of heart attack and stroke; offers heart-healthy lifestyle tips and tools; and sponsors a program called the Heart of Diabetes, which provides information on how diabetes increases the risk of heart disease and stroke.

> American Heart Association
> National Center
> 7272 Greenville Ave.
> Dallas, TX 75231
> 1-800-242-8721
> www.americanheart.org

American Obesity Association: An organization for advocacy and education on obesity. Provides information on prevention, treatment, consumer protection, and discrimination.

> American Obesity Association
> 1250 24th St., NW, Suite 300
> Washington, D.C. 20037
> 1-202-776-7711
> www.obesity.org

Body mass index calculator: A tool sponsored by the National Heart, Lung, and Blood Institute of the National Institutes of Health. Go to www.nhlbisupport.com/bmi and plug in your height and weight. The program will calculate your BMI and tell you what it means.

Centers for Disease Control and Prevention: A government organization that collects statistical data and identifies trends; features general information about diabetes, prevention, and care; sponsors public-awareness campaigns; and publishes such reports as "Diabetes and Women's Health across Life Stages: A Public Health Perspective," "A National Public Health Initiative on Diabetes and Women's Health," National Diabetes Fact Sheet, and "Take Charge of Your Diabetes," a patient guide. Also available online: Wisewoman Program, which includes resources for women on heart disease and lowering risk (www.cdc.gov/wisewoman.resources.htm).

> Centers for Disease Control and Prevention
> National Center for Chronic Disease Prevention and Health Promotion
> (toll-free) 1-877-CDC-DIAB (877-232-3422)
> www.cdc.gov/diabetes
> email: diabetes@cdc.gov

Diabetes Prevention Program: Clinical trial that showed lifestyle changes in diet and exercise could significantly delay or prevent diabetes. General information about this clinical trial and its results can be found at www.bsc.gwu.edu/dpp/index.htmlvdoc with a link to the lifestyle manuals used by participants in the program to lose weight and get active. These include handouts you can download on such topics as "Be a Fat Detective," "Take Charge of What's around You," "You Can Manage Stress," and "Ways to Stay Motivated."

National Diabetes Information Clearinghouse (NDIC): A service of the National Institute of Diabetes and Digestive and Kidney Disease, National Institutes of Health. The NDIC develops and distributes free publications about diabetes; provides information about treatments, diabetes complications, clinical trials, paying for care, finding health professionals, and other diabetes topics; and responds to public inquiries about diabetes.

> NDIC
> 1 Information Way
> Bethesda, MD 20892-3560
> 1-800-860-8747
> http://diabetes.niddk.nih.gov
> email: ndic@info.niddk.nih.gov

The NDIC also sponsors:

Weight-Control Information Network: A source of "up-to-date, science-based information on weight control, obesity, physical activity, and related nutritional topics." Produces such booklets as "Active at Any Size" and "Choosing a Safe and Successful Weight Loss Program."

> Weight-Control Information Network
> 1 WIN Way
> Bethesda, MD 20892-3665
> (toll-free) 1-877-946-4627
> http://win.niddk.nih.gov
> email: win@info.niddk.nih.gov

The National Women's Health Information Center: A service of the Office on Women's Health, U.S. Department of Health and Human Services. A website and toll-free phone number, which provides free, reliable health information on more than one hundred health topics of interest to women.

> 1-800-994-WOMAN
> www.4women.gov

Appendixes

Appendix 1

Body Mass Index (BMI) Table

BMI	Normal						Overweight					Obese				
height (inches)	19	20	21	22	23	24	25	26	27	28	29	30	31	32	33	34
							Body weight (pounds)									
58	91	96	100	105	110	115	119	124	129	134	138	143	148	153	158	162
59	94	99	104	109	114	119	124	128	133	138	143	148	153	158	163	168
60	97	102	107	112	118	123	128	133	138	143	148	153	158	163	168	174
61	100	106	111	116	122	127	132	137	143	148	153	158	164	169	174	180
62	104	109	115	120	126	131	136	142	147	153	158	164	169	175	180	186
63	107	113	118	124	130	135	141	146	152	158	163	169	175	180	186	191
64	110	116	122	128	134	140	145	151	157	163	169	174	180	186	192	197
65	114	120	126	132	138	144	150	156	162	168	174	180	186	192	198	204
66	118	124	130	136	142	148	155	161	167	173	179	186	192	198	204	210
67	121	127	134	140	146	153	159	166	172	178	185	191	198	204	211	217
68	125	131	138	144	151	158	164	171	177	184	190	197	203	210	216	223
69	128	135	142	149	155	162	169	176	182	189	196	203	209	216	223	230
70	132	139	146	153	160	167	174	181	188	195	202	209	216	222	229	236
71	136	143	150	157	165	172	179	186	193	200	208	215	222	229	236	243
72	140	147	154	162	169	177	184	191	199	206	213	221	228	235	242	250
73	144	151	159	166	174	182	189	197	204	212	219	227	235	242	250	257
74	148	155	163	171	179	186	194	202	210	218	225	233	241	249	256	264
75	152	160	168	176	184	192	200	208	216	224	232	240	248	256	264	272
76	156	164	172	180	189	197	205	213	221	230	238	246	254	263	271	279

BMI is a general indicator of body weight. The higher your BMI, the greater your risk of developing diabetes, high blood pressure, and heart disease.

	Obese					Extreme obesity												
BMI height (inches)	35	36	37	38	39	40	41	42	43	44	45	46	47	48	49	50	51	52
						Body weight (pounds)												
58	167	172	177	181	186	191	196	201	205	210	215	220	224	229	234	239	244	248
59	173	178	183	188	193	198	203	208	212	217	222	227	232	237	242	247	252	257
60	179	184	189	194	199	204	209	215	220	225	230	235	240	245	250	255	261	266
61	185	190	195	201	206	211	217	222	227	232	238	243	248	254	259	264	269	275
62	191	196	202	207	213	218	224	229	235	240	246	251	256	262	267	273	278	284
63	197	203	208	214	220	225	231	237	242	248	254	259	265	270	276	282	287	293
64	204	209	215	221	227	232	238	244	250	256	262	267	273	279	285	291	296	302
65	210	216	222	228	234	240	246	252	258	264	270	276	282	288	294	300	306	312
66	216	223	229	235	241	247	253	260	266	272	278	284	291	297	303	309	315	322
67	223	230	236	242	249	255	261	268	274	280	287	293	299	306	312	319	325	331
68	230	236	243	249	256	262	269	276	282	289	295	302	308	315	322	328	335	341
69	236	243	250	257	263	270	277	284	291	297	304	311	318	324	331	338	345	351
70	243	250	257	264	271	278	285	292	299	306	313	320	327	334	341	348	355	362
71	250	257	265	272	279	286	293	301	308	315	322	329	336	343	351	358	365	372
72	258	265	272	279	287	294	302	309	316	324	331	338	346	353	361	368	375	383
73	265	272	280	288	295	302	310	318	325	333	340	348	355	363	371	378	386	393
74	272	280	287	295	303	311	319	326	334	342	350	358	365	373	381	389	396	404
75	279	287	295	303	311	319	327	335	343	351	359	367	375	383	391	399	407	415
76	287	295	304	312	320	328	336	344	353	361	369	377	385	394	402	410	418	426

Source: "Body Mass Index Table," National Heart, Lung, and Blood Institute (www.nhlbi.nih.gov/guidelines/obesity/bmi_tbl.htm).

Appendix 2

Carbohydrate Counts for Common Fruits, Vegetables, Starches, and Dairy

Fruits and vegetables

Foods	Serving size	Carbohydrates (grams)
Canned green beans	1/2 cup	4
Broccoli	1 cup	5
Carrots	1/2 cup	4
Cucumber	1 cup	3
Lettuce	1 cup	1
Spinach	1 cup	2
Tomatoes	1 cup	8
Small apple	1	16
Small banana	1	16
Grapes	17	15
Orange	1 medium	15
Unsweetened applesauce	1/2 cup	14
Apple juice	1/2 cup	13
Orange juice	1/2 cup	13

Starches

Foods	Serving size	Carbohydrates (grams)
Bagel	1/2 (35 grams)	19
Whole-wheat bread	1 slice	13
White bread	1 slice	12
English muffin	1/2	13
Tortilla	1	12
Cheerios	3/4 cup	16
Cornflakes	3/4 cup	20
Raisin Bran	1/2 cup	22
Plain oatmeal	1/2 cup cooked	13
Graham crackers	3	16
Popcorn	3 cups	11
Pretzels	3/4 oz.	17
Tortilla chips	17	18
White rice	1/3 cup cooked	15
Brown rice	1/3 cup cooked	15

Starches *(continued)*

Foods	Serving size	Carbohydrates (grams)
Macaroni	1/2 cup cooked	20
Spaghetti	1/2 cup cooked	20
Baked beans	1/3 cup cooked	17
Garbanzo beans	1/2 cup cooked	22
Lentil beans	1/2 cup cooked	20
Canned corn	1/2 cup cooked	20
Peas	1/2 cup cooked	11
Baked potato	3 oz.	22
Mashed potato	1/2 cup	16

Dairy

Foods	Serving size	Carbohydrates (grams)
Milk, any kind	1 cup	11
Nonfat yogurt	3/4 cup	13
Low-fat yogurt with fruit	1 cup	47
Tofu	1/2 cup	2
American cheese	1 slice	2
Cottage cheese	1/4 cup	3

Source: Hope S. Warshaw and Karmeen Kulkarni, *Complete Guide to Carb Counting* (American Diabetes Association), 2001.

Appendix 3

Sample Grocery List for Healthful Eating

Try to create your own grocery list, marking items to avoid, those to eat in small quantities, and good items to include in your diet. On the next page you'll find one example of a grocery list. The American Diabetes Association has created a "virtual grocery store" at http://vgs.diabetes.org/grocery_tour.jsp to help you create your own shopping list.

GROCERY LIST Mark the list with: X = items to avoid ↔ = those you can eat, but in small quantities ☺ = good items to include in your diet

☺ Fresh produce	Juices/Snacks	Deli/Bakery	Dairy
Apples	X ANY fruit juice	↔ Roast beef	☺ Milk, 1%, 2%, or skim
Bananas	☺ Applesauce, preferably natural	↔ Turkey breast, try low fat	☺ Yogurt, plain, low or nonfat
Blueberries	☺ Applesauce, snack size	↔ Bologna, low fat	↔ Butter, Land O'Lakes lightly salted
Cantaloupe	X Doritos, potato chips, cheese puffs, tortilla	↔ Salami	↔ Sour cream, low fat
Carrots	chips	↔ Ham	X Cream
Celery	☺ Popcorn	**Meat**	↔ Eggs, brown or white
Corn	**Tomato sauce/soup**	X Bacon	↔ Processed cheese, low fat
Cucumbers	☺ Tomato sauce (check sugar content)	↔ Chopped hamburger, try low fat	↔ Cream cheese, low fat
Eggplant	☺ Progresso canned tomatoes	↔ Beef stew, try low fat	☺ Simply Smart or Lactaid milk
Garlic	↔ Tomato paste	☺ Turkey	**Frozen**
Ginger	☺ Chicken broth	☺ Chicken	↔ Check labels on any processed frozen food
Leeks	☺ Processed soups (check labels)	☺ Pork	☺ Any plain frozen vegetables
Lettuce	☺ Canned tuna, preferably in water	↔ Hotdogs	↔ Ice cream (check labels)
Mushrooms	**Rice/pasta**	**Bread**	
Onions	↔ White rice	↔ White (wheat is better)	
Raspberries	↔ Brown long-grain rice	X Bagels	
Scallions	↔ Couscous	↔ Pita or lavash	
Shallots	↔ Pasta	**Cookies and snack cakes**	
Spinach	**Cereals**	X Avoid this group altogether; if you have to buy,	
Snow Peas	X High-sugar cereals (check labels)	choose low-fat variety	
Squash	↔ Cheerios	↔ Crackers (check labels)	
Strawberries	↔ Life	**Baking**	
Sweet potatoes	↔ Corn flakes	↔ Sugar, preferably brown	
Tomatoes	☺ Quaker Instant Oatmeal, preferably regular	↔ Flour, preferably wheat	
White potatoes	X Cereal bars	☺ Peanut butter	
Watermelon	X PopTarts	↔ Any jellies, preserves, or jam	
Zucchini	↔ Granola bars (check labels)		
↔ **Dried fruit, including raisins**			

Appendix 4

Choosing a Blood Glucose Meter

➡ When choosing a blood glucose meter, consider ease of use, speed, and size, but bear in mind that consistency and accuracy are the most important features. Your diabetes nurse educator may have some good suggestions for reliable meters.

➡ Many glucose meters are provided free of charge by the manufacturer. (Companies usually make their profits on the strips, rather than on the machine itself.) Also, some health plans only cover certain models of blood glucose meters and strips, so check with your health insurance company before you head out to purchase a meter.

➡ Talk to other people with diabetes about which meters they use and why.

➡ If you want to track your results electronically, choose a model that is compatible with software that can download the results to a computer or PDA.

➡ If you live in an extreme climate or high altitude, find out if your choice of model has a temperature or altitude range limit.

➡ Buyer beware: Check the web for up-to-date notice of medical device recalls. Two models rated "best" by a national consumer organization in 2005 were later recalled.

➡ Large displays and "talking" models are available for users with visual impairments.

➡ Most models use test strips that cost between $1,000 and $1,300 annually. Most medical insurance companies and HMOs cover the cost of strips, so you will be responsible only for a small co-payment. However, check with your insurance company first, as your choice may be limited to a few approved models.

Types of Meters

Type	Representative manufacturers/brands	Pros and cons to consider
Traditional battery-operated meters	Most major brands	Use individual test strips or a drum of strips. Most models are under $100, lightweight, and offer quick, accurate test results with a minuscule blood sample. They often have a memory function to store results.

Type	Representative manufacturers/brands	Pros and cons to consider
Blood glucose meter, available with remote connection to the Medtronic MiniMed insulin pump	Paradigm (Becton Dickinson and Medtronic MiniMed insulin pump)	Monitor sends wireless reading to pump; patient can use data to adjust insulin dose. Manufacturer offers patients online management of their data.
Disposable meters	NewTek (ReliOn)	Models priced under $60 come preloaded with 100 test strips. Available at Wal-Mart, which owns the ReliOn brand.
Diabetes management software	Bayer Ascensia, Freestyle, Lifescan, and others	Monitor can download readings to PDA, cell phone, or computer. Offers diabetes management and log-keeping via software. Some software can also help with management of insulin pumps.
Noninvasive monitors	Newly approved models (CGMS System Gold by Medtronic MiniMed; DexCom STS) provide continuous glucose monitoring via a patch—no blood is drawn. Monitor must be calibrated with three or four fingerstick tests per day.	Continuously monitors glucose levels for up to three days. Alarm alerts wearer to dangerously high or low glucose levels. Additional data may help doctor tailor treatment plan. May not be accurate in low blood sugar range.

Features of Blood Glucose Meters

Blood glucose meter	Multisite	Sample size (microliters)	Memory	Test time	Comments
LifeScan					
• One Touch Basic	no	10	75	45 secs.	Software available on all products
• One Touch FastTake	no	1.5	150 tests	15 secs.	
• One Touch SureStep	no	10	150 tests	15 secs.	Easy to use if you have problems with arthritis or manual dexterity.
• One Touch Ultra	yes	1.0	150 tests	5 secs.	
• One Touch UltraSmart	yes	1.0	150 tests	5 secs.	

Blood glucose meter	Multisite	Sample size (microliters)	Memory	Test time	Comments
Abbott					
• FreeStyle Flash	yes	0.3	250 tests	15 secs.	Smallest blood glucose meter
• FreeStyle	yes	0.3	250 tests	7 secs.	
Roche Diagnostics					
• AccuChek Compact	yes	1.5	100 tests	8 secs.	Has an automatic drum that calibrates meter for you
• AccuChek Advantage/ Voicemate	no	3.0	480 tests	26 secs.	System that talks to you. Designed for the sight impaired. Easy to use if you have problems with arthritis or manual dexterity.
Bayer Diagnostics					
• Ascensia Breeze	yes	3.0	100 tests	30 secs.	Has a ten-strip autodisc so you don't have to handle strips. Meter requires no coding. Software available.
• Ascensia Contour	yes	0.6	240 tests	15 secs.	Software available
Becton Dickinson Diabetes					
• BD Logic	no	0.3	250 tests	5 secs.	Software available
Hypoguard					
• Advance Intuition	no	3.0	10 tests	10 secs.	Large display screen. Software available.
• ReliOn New Tek	no	3.0	100 preloaded strips	15 secs.	Available only at Wal-Mart. Disposable.
• ReliOn Ultima	No	3.0	450 tests	15 secs.	Available only at Wal-Mart

Note: Websites that regularly review blood glucose meters include www.diabetes.org (American Diabetes Association), www.childrenwithdiabetes.com, www.diabetesnet.com, and www.consumerreports.org.

Source: Adapted from Diabetes Mall, Health through Information website: www.diabetesnet.com, 2004, and American Diabetes Association website: www.diabetes.org, Resource Guide 2005.

Appendix 5

Mixing Different Kinds of Insulin

If your medical provider recommends that you mix a rapid-acting or very rapid–acting insulin with an intermediate-acting insulin, follow the instructions below (review them with your health care team first). Note that the insulins Lantus (glargine) and Levamir (detemir) cannot be mixed with other insulins.

➡ Start with the long-acting, cloudy insulin. Gently roll the vial between your hands to mix it up.

➡ Wipe the top of the bottles with an alcohol prep.

➡ Pull back the plunger of the syringe to the dose of longer-acting insulin (you will see air in the syringe).

➡ Keep the vial upright on the table and inject the air into the longer-acting, cloudy insulin bottle. Then remove the needle, but don't draw up insulin.

➡ Pull back on the plunger of the syringe to the dose of short-acting, clear insulin (again, you will have air in the syringe).

➡ Inject the air into the short-acting (clear) insulin bottle, and then turn the bottle upside down and withdraw your dose of clear insulin.

➡ Return to the longer-acting, cloudy insulin bottle. Turn it upside down, insert the needle so it is in the insulin, then slowly pull the plunger back to measure your total dose.

➡ Always draw up the clear insulin before the cloudy when mixing insulin.

Source: Adapted from Kathy Hurxthal, *An Introduction to Diabetes* (Diabetes Center, Massachusetts General Hospital, 2002).

Appendix 6

Disposing of Syringes

Syringes are medical waste and need to be disposed of carefully. Store all used syringes in a container that can be tightly sealed. Available products include:

➡ BD Home Sharps Container (BD Consumer Healthcare)
➡ BD Safe Clip (Becton Dickenson Consumer Products)
➡ MED-SAFE Insulin and Lancet Disposal System (Med-Safe Systems)
➡ GRP Medical Services mail-back sharps disposal program
➡ Voyager Diabetic Needle Disposal

Remember, you can reuse needles, but you should discard any that are dirty, blunt, or worn.

For more information on needle disposal, contact your local American Diabetes Association affiliate, the Center for Disease Control (www.cdc.gov), or Diabetes 123 at www.diabetes123.com.

Appendix 7

Insulin Pumps and Other Insulin Delivery Systems

Type of insulin delivery system	Mechanism of delivery	Comments
Insulin syringes	Draw up insulin into syringe and then inject needle under skin.	Least expensive method. Available in both short and long needles and various volumes (3/10 cc, 1/2 cc, and 1 cc). Used with 10 cc insulin bottles that hold a total of 1,000 units. May be difficult for some people to read measurement markings on syringe.
Insulin pens	Store insulin in a pen cartridge and then inject with pen needle under skin.	Pens come as completely disposable or with disposable cartridges. You select your dose of insulin using a dial on the pen. The pen needles are disposable and are available in a variety of sizes.
Insulin jet injectors	Inject insulin through skin with air pressure.	There are no needles. Injectors can cause bruising and are difficult to use. Require frequent cleaning. Not often recommended.
Insulin pump	Looks like a pager. Stores rapid- or very rapid–acting insulin that is delivered continuously through a plastic catheter.	May be easier for those with type 1 diabetes on intensive insulin therapy (4 or more injections/day). Expensive. Requires training and frequent blood glucose monitoring, as well as the ability to program the pump. Not usually used in type 2 diabetes.
Inhaled insulin	Breathe rapid-acting insulin in through an inhaler	Approved in 2006

Source: Adapted from Kathy Hurxthal, *An Introduction to Diabetes* (Diabetes Center, Massachusetts General Hospital, 2002).

Insulin pump companies

Company	Website
Medtronic MiniMed	www.minimed.com
Disetronic	www.disetronic-usa.com
Animas	www.animascorp.com
DANA Diabecare	www.danapumps.com

Appendix 8

Over-the-Counter Medications and Diabetes

Types of medication	Medications that are generally safe for someone with diabetes	Medications to use with caution
Cough medications	Cepacol sugar-free tablets Cerose DM expectorant	Cough syrups with sucrose pseudoephedrine Decongestants with Robitussin
Fever reducers	Tylenol Aspirin	Prolonged use of non-steroidal anti-inflammatories (NSAIDs) such as ibuprofen and naproxen (e.g., Motrin, Aleve) may cause kidney damage.
Antidiarrheal medications	Kaopectate Pepto Bismol	

Appendix 9

Complementary (Alternative Medicine) Treatments

Western medical science is just beginning to evaluate rigorously herbal and traditional medicines used around the world. At this point they are all considered to be unproven therapies. It is important for you to mention to your health care providers if you are taking or are planning to take any herbal or vitamin/mineral supplements so they can be alert to side effects or interactions with other medications you are taking.

Physicians affiliated with Harvard Medical School's Division for Research and Education in Complementary and Integrative Medical Therapies have conducted a review of all the scientific literature published in English that relates to the safety of herbal therapies and vitamin/mineral supplements for people with diabetes. They assessed the quality of the evidence on thirty-six herbs and nine vitamin/minerals using criteria or scales that have been scientifically validated.

On the basis of their analyses, they identified the seven herbs and vitamin/mineral supplements listed below as the most promising at this time. However, they also point out that there isn't enough evidence to recommend or discourage use of any one supplement in particular.

Best evidence, but not conclusive:

Plant	Description	Comments
Coccinia indica (ivy gourd)	Plant that grows wild on India subcontinent; powder from crushed leaves given in tablet or pellet form	Evidence from two high-quality controlled clinical trials shows blood-glucose–lowering effect and warrants further study
American ginseng	Ground root taken in capsule form; American species most studied, but also includes Chinese, Korean, Japanese, and Siberian species	Studies suggest possible glucose-lowering effect of American species, but larger studies and longer-term follow-up needed

Evidence that suggests benefit but needs more study:

Plant	Description	Comment
Momordica charantia	Vegetable indigenous to tropical areas; given in injectable extracts, fruit juice, or as melon bits	Limited data but results suggest a potential effect for diabetes
Opuntia streptacantha (nopal)	Prickly pear cactus found in arid regions in Western hemisphere; used for glucose control by those of Mexican descent	Most trials published in Spanish; those in English suggest enhanced insulin sensitivity, but longer-term clinical trials are needed
L-carnitine	Given intravenously (no studies yet of orally given preparations)	Cellular studies suggest its role in free fatty acid and glucose oxidation; clinical data are limited but promising
Gymnema sylvestre	Plant found in tropical India, commonly used as leaf extract in Ayurveda (East Indian healing system)	Limited data that are suggestive but inconclusive as far as effect on blood glucose
Aloe vera	Desert plant popularly used to treat burns; given in juice form	Data are preliminary but suggest a potential glucose-lowering effect
vanadium	a nutrient that is either nonessential or required only in minute amounts	Suggestive results on glucose control, but no randomized controlled studies have been done. Salt form caused some gastrointestinal discomfort, but less discomfort if given in an organically chelated compound.

Source: Adapted from G.Y. Yeh et al., "Systematic Review of Herbs and Dietary Supplements for Glycemic Control in Diabetes," *Diabetes Care,* 26(4), 2003. Can be found online at http://care.diabetesjournals.org/cgi/content/full/26/4/1277.

Appendix 10

Your Diabetic Targets

Daily glucose testing (whole blood value mg/dl)

Before meals	80–120
1 to 2 hours after start of a meal	140–180
Before bed	100–140

Hemoglobin A_{1c}

Lab test checked every 3 months in doctor's office	less than 7 percent

Cholesterol

Total cholesterol	<200 mg/dl
HDL cholesterol	>50 mg/dl
LDL cholesterol	<100 mg/dl (if not lower)
Triglycerides	<150mg/dl

Blood pressure

Measured 3 separate days same time of the day at home and once a year during a visit to the doctor's office	<130/80

Other tests/vaccinations

Annual urine sample for microalbumin	<30 mg per gram of creatinine
Annual eye examination with eye specialist	
Foot examination at every visit	
Annual influenza vaccination	
Pneumococcal pneumonia vaccination every 10 years	

Lifestyle changes

Take an aspirin a day
Exercise at least 3–4 times per week
Make healthy food choices
Quit smoking
Reduce stress

Glossary of Terms

Acidosis: See *Diabetic ketoacidosis.*

Activities of daily living: Scale developed by S. Katz and colleagues to measure personal self-maintenance ability among older adults. The activities rated are eating, toileting, dressing, bathing, transferring (e.g., getting in and out of bed), and continence.

Adherence: The extent to which patients follow health care provider recommendations for disease management, including health-promoting activities. For people with diabetes, this includes taking medications, monitoring blood glucose, and following nutrition and physical activity guidelines. Also see *Compliance.*

Adiposity: Excessive fat in the body. Also see *Obesity.*

Age-adjusted: Describes rates that have been adjusted by an established procedure to minimize the effects of differences in age composition when comparing rates for different populations.

Albuminuria: More than normal amounts of the protein albumin in the urine. Albuminuria may be a sign of kidney disease.

American Diabetes Association (ADA): Nonprofit national health organization that provides information, advocates policy change, and conducts research to prevent and cure diabetes and to improve the life of all people affected by diabetes. For more information, see www.diabetes.org.

Angina: A condition in which the heart muscle does not receive enough blood, resulting in pain in the chest.

Angiotensin converting enzyme (ACE) inhibitor: A type of drug used to lower blood pressure and to help prevent progression of kidney disease in people with diabetes.

Anorexia: Lack or loss of appetite for food.

Anorexia nervosa: A serious eating disorder characterized by chronic decreased food intake that results in profound weight loss.

Atherosclerosis/atherosclerotic disease: A disease in which fat builds up in the large and medium-sized arteries. This build-up of fat may slow down or stop blood flow. People with diabetes are at increased risk for atherosclerosis.

Atherosclerotic lesions/plaque: Deposits in the arteries that result from the accumulation of cholesterol and lipids in the arteries.

Autonomic neuropathy: Nerve damage affecting control of the internal organs, such as the bladder muscles, digestive tract, heart, and genital organs. Autonomic neuropathy can develop as a complication of diabetes.

Basal insulin: A component of insulin therapy (along with bolus insulin) meant to maintain a stable level of insulin throughout the day and night.

Beta cell: Type of cell in the pancreas that makes and releases insulin.

Body mass index (BMI): A measure of body size that relates weight to height. Formula: weight in kilograms divided by height in meters squared. BMI correlates highly with body fat in most people.

Bolus insulin: The dose of insulin given before meals that is calculated to keep blood glucose levels under control (usually less than 180 mg/dl) after meals. The dose changes on the basis of meal size and composition, blood glucose level at the time, and anticipated exercise after the meal.

Bulimia: Eating disorder characterized by binge eating and induced vomiting.

Cardiovascular disease (CVD): Disease of the circulatory system, including the heart and blood vessels. Diabetes increases the risk of CVD two- to fivefold.

Cataract: Clouding of the lens of the eye. Diabetes increases the occurrence of cataracts.

Central adiposity or obesity: Fat deposits that form in the center of a person's body, especially around the intestines, often assessed by measuring waist-to-hip ratio. Central adiposity increases the risk of cardiovascular complications.

Cerebrovascular disease: Damage to the blood vessels supplying the brain that can result in a stroke (see *Stroke*). Diabetes increases the risk of stroke two-fold.

Cholesterol: A fatlike substance in the blood, muscle, liver, brain, and other tissues. Too much cholesterol may cause fat to build up in the artery walls and cause disease that slows or stops the flow of blood.

Clinical trials: Human research studies designed to produce statistically valid information on how best to treat patients.

Comorbidity: The condition of having more than one illness at the same time (e.g., diabetes and depression, diabetes and heart disease).

Compliance: Patients' adherence to health care provider recommendations for disease management and health-promoting activities. See also *Adherence.*

Complications of diabetes: The chronic (long-term) effects of diabetes resulting in diseases of the eyes, kidneys, nerves, and circulatory system, which carries blood to the heart, brain, and limbs. The development of these complications is related to the duration of diabetes, levels of blood glucose over time, and other factors, such as blood pressure levels and genetics.

Coronary heart disease (CHD): Destruction and weakening of heart muscle, secondary to decreased blood supply (atherosclerosis). The most serious danger of coronary heart disease is a heart attack, which occurs when the supply of blood to the heart is greatly reduced or stopped due to a blockage in a coronary artery. People with diabetes are two to five times more likely to have CHD than those without diabetes.

Cortisol: One of several hormones made in the adrenal glands. Cortisol is one of the main hormones secreted as part of the stress response; it can raise blood glucose levels.

Dementia: Loss of cognitive function; a condition of deteriorated mentality.

Dentition: Quality and quantity of teeth, including their number, kind, and arrangement.

Diabetes Control and Complications Trial (DCCT): Clinical study funded by the National Institutes of Health to assess the effects of intensive therapy on the long-term complications of type 1 diabetes. The study showed that intensive blood glucose control slows the onset and progression of eye, kidney, and nerve disease caused by diabetes. For more information, see www.niddk.nih.gov/health/diabetes/pubs/dcct1/dcct.htm.

Diabetes Prevention Program (DPP): Clinical trial sponsored by the National Institutes of Health that compared the effectiveness of diet and exercise with that of metformin or a placebo in reducing the risk for type 2 diabetes in high-risk people. For more information, see www.bsc.gwu.edu/dpp/index.htmlvdoc.

Diabetes risk profile: A descriptive term for a person's level of known risk factors for diabetes (e.g., body mass index, physical activity level, family history).

Diabetic ketoacidosis: Acute complication of diabetes characterized by high blood glucose in the presence of ketones in the urine and bloodstream. Diabetic ketoacidosis is often caused by illness or taking too little insulin. It requires emergency treatment. Symptoms include nausea and vomiting, stomach pain, and deep, rapid breathing.

Dyslipidemia: Abnormal excess or abnormal forms of fat or lipids in the blood.

Dyslipoproteinemia: Abnormal concentrations of one or more lipoproteins, a combination of a lipid and a protein, used to transport cholesterol and other lipids through the bloodstream.

Early Treatment of Diabetic Retinopathy Study (ETDRS): Study that examined the effects of laser photocoagulation or aspirin on the progression of diabetic retinopathy in patients with diabetes. For more information, see www.nei.nih.gov/neitrials_static/study53.htm.

Eclampsia: Severe hypertension accompanied by seizures. Considered an obstetric emergency requiring immediate caesarean section.

Edentulous: Describes the loss of teeth, especially in elderly people; toothless.

End-stage kidney disease (ESKD): The final phase of kidney disease, requiring treatment with dialysis or kidney transplantation. ESKD can be a complication of diabetes.

Epinephrine: Principal blood pressure–raising hormone secreted by the adrenal medulla. Also released under times of stress.

Estrogen replacement therapy (ERT): Refers to the use of estrogen as a prescription drug to replace the hormone estrogen, which is no longer produced by the ovaries as a result of menopause.

Excess mortality: Increased rates or numbers of deaths in a specific population by age, sex, cause, and sometimes other variables.

Fasting glucose: Glucose concentration in a person who has not eaten recently (usually for at least eight hours); used to diagnose diabetes.

Fatalism: A belief that events are predetermined and cannot be altered by human effect.

Fetal malformations: Abnormalities in the heart, urinary tract, digestive tract, spinal cord, or limbs present at birth. High levels of glucose can pass from mother to baby and affect the baby's early organ development in the first six to eight weeks of pregnancy, resulting in malformations. This is why tight control of blood glucose is critical before conception.

Free fatty acids: Circulating fats in the blood. Though free fatty acids are a necessary source of fuel for the body, too much of them contributes to insulin resistance and may also lead to atherosclerosis, a process that narrows blood vessels to the heart and brain. Most obese people have high levels of free fatty acids in their blood.

Functional impairment: Damage that affects a person's ability to perform daily activities.

Gangrene: Death of body tissue as a result of poor circulation. Gangrene is a serious complication of diabetes and may lead to amputation.

Gestational diabetes mellitus (GDM): Type of diabetes that can occur during pregnancy; in most cases, blood sugar levels return to normal after pregnancy. Affects 3 to 5 percent of all pregnancies.

Glaucoma: Eye disease associated with increased pressure within the eye that can damage the optic nerve and cause impaired vision and blindness. People with diabetes are at increased risk of glaucoma.

Glomerular filtration rate: Measure of the kidney's ability to filter and remove waste products; used to diagnose kidney disease.

Glucose tolerance test: A kind of stress test used to diagnose diabetes. Blood glucose is measured before a patient has eaten that day. Blood is subsequently tested after the patient drinks a liquid containing glucose to see how the patient's body metabolizes glucose over time. A more sensitive method of diagnosing diabetes and prediabetes than fasting tests.

Glycated hemoglobin: See *Hemoglobin A_{1c}.*

Glycemic control: The level of glucose in the blood or, for the measurement of chronic control, the level of hemoglobin A_{1c}.

Glycosuria: The presence of glucose in the urine, a sign of poor blood glucose control.

Glycosylated hemoglobin test: See *Hemoglobin A_{1c}.*

HDL cholesterol: High-density lipoprotein cholesterol, a transport form of cholesterol in the blood. Low concentrations of HDL cholesterol are a risk factor for cardiovascular disease (CVD), especially in people with diabetes; high levels are protective.

Hemoglobin A_{1c} (HgbA$_{1c}$): A blood test that measures a person's average blood glucose level for the two- to three-month period before the test.

Hormone replacement therapy (HRT): Refers to the use of hormones as prescription drugs to replace the hormones estrogen and progesterone, which women's ovaries stop producing during menopause. (See *Estrogen Replacement Therapy.*)

Hypercholesterolemia: Abnormally high levels of cholesterol in the blood.

Hyperglycemia: High levels of glucose (sugar) in the blood, a hallmark of diabetes. Hyperglycemia occurs when the body does not have enough insulin or cannot use the insulin it does have to transport glucose into cells. Signs of hyperglycemia include increased thirst, dry mouth, and a need to urinate often.

Hyperinsulinemia: A high level of insulin in the blood. Increased levels of insulin often indicate underlying insulin resistance. (See *Insulin resistance.*)

Hyperlipidemia: Too high a level of fats (lipids) in the blood.

Hyperosmolar coma: Loss of consciousness or altered mental status (confusion or drowsiness) related to very high levels of glucose in the blood. Requires emergency treatment.

Hypertension: High blood pressure, a condition that occurs when vessel resistance is high and blood circulates through the arteries with too much force, increasing the risk of heart attack, stroke, diabetic eye complications, and kidney problems.

Hypertriglyceridemia: A high level of triglycerides, a type of blood fat. Triglycerides can increase when diabetes and weight are not under control.

Hypoglycemia: A condition that occurs in people with diabetes when their blood glucose levels are too low, usually less than 65 mg/dl. Symptoms include anxiety or confusion, a rapid heart rate, trembling, and sweating. If not treated promptly, more severe effects can occur, including confusion, coma, or seizures.

Hypoglycemic agent: Drug used to treat hyperglycemia in people with diabetes.

Impaired fasting glucose (IFG): A fasting plasma glucose equal to or greater than 100 mg/dl and less than 126 mg/dl. IFG is one form of prediabetes, a risk factor for future diabetes.

Impaired glucose tolerance (IGT): A plasma glucose level between 140 and 200 mg/dl two hours after a seventy-five-gram oral glucose tolerance test. IGT is a form of prediabetes, a risk factor for the development of future diabetes and cardiovascular disease.

Incidence: The number of new cases of a disease among a certain group of people during a certain period of time.

Insulin: A hormone normally secreted by the beta cells of the pancreas. Insulin controls the level of glucose (sugar) in the blood.

Insulin pump: A device that delivers a continuous supply of insulin into the body (also called continuous subcutaneous insulin infusion). The insulin is pumped through a plastic tube that is connected to a needle, which is inserted into the skin. Insulin is delivered at one or more steady rates (called basal rates) for continuous daylong coverage, with extra boosts of insulin (called boluses) to cover meals or other times when extra insulin is needed.

Insulin resistance: Abnormal metabolic state in which cells lose sensitivity to insulin. Insulin resistance is an underlying factor in the development of type 2 diabetes; it also increases risk of cardiovascular disease.

Intensive glucose control: Diabetes management aimed at maintaining glucose levels as close to the nondiabetic range as safely possible, compensating for meals, activity level, menstruation, stress, and illness. Intensive or "tight" control has been shown to prevent or at least delay many of the medical complications of diabetes.

Ischemic heart disease: See *Coronary heart disease.*

Juvenile Diabetes Research Foundation International (JDRF): Major diabetes organization focused exclusively on diabetes research. JDRF focuses on type 1 diabetes. For more information, see www.jdf.org.

Ketoacidosis: See *Diabetic ketoacidosis.*

LDL cholesterol: Low-density lipoprotein cholesterol, a transport form of cholesterol in the blood. High concentrations of LDL cholesterol are a risk factor for cardiovascular disease.

Lipids: Fats, including cholesterol, triglycerides, and phospholipids.

Lipoprotein: Combination of protein and fat that transports lipids (cholesterol, triglycerides) in the bloodstream. Major lipoproteins are named for their density and buoyancy in water, such as low-density (LDL), high-density (HDL), and very low–density (VLDL) lipoproteins.

Locus of control: A common measure of a person's perceived ability to control events.

Macroalbuminuria: High levels of the protein albumin in urine, a sign of progressing kidney disease. Usually greater than 300 mg per twenty-four hours.

Macrosomia: A condition in which a baby is "large-for-date," that is, weighs more than normal as a result of high blood glucose levels. Macrosomia can complicate the delivery.

Macrovascular disease: Disease of the large blood vessels caused by atherosclerosis. There are three types of macrovascular disease: coronary (heart) disease, cerebrovascular disease (vessels supplying the brain), and peripheral vascular disease (vessels supplying the extremities).

Metabolism: The chemical and physical processes in the body that sustain life and are related to the assimilation of food, growth, and provision of energy. Diabetes affects many aspects of the body's metabolism.

Metformin: A drug used to treat type 2 diabetes.

mg/dl: Milligrams per deciliter. Term used to describe how much of a substance is in a specific amount of liquid (e.g., the number of milligrams of glucose in one deciliter of blood).

Microalbuminuria: Low but abnormal levels of albumin excretion in the urine. Microalbuminuria is defined as more than 30 mg of the protein albumin excreted in a twenty-four-hour period or as a spot urine sample with 30 mg per gram of creatinine. It is an early indicator and risk factor for future kidney disease.

Microvascular disease: Disease of the small blood vessels, especially of the kidney or the eye.

Myocardial infarction (MI): Also called a heart attack, MI occurs when heart muscle is destroyed as a result of narrowed or blocked blood vessels that interrupt the blood supply to the area. MI is a serious complication of diabetes that can cause death.

National Cholesterol Education Program (NCEP): Program begun in 1985 by the National Institutes of Health. The goal is to reduce the percentage of Americans with high blood cholesterol through educational efforts. The NCEP raises awareness of high blood cholesterol as a risk factor for coronary heart disease and teaches the benefits of lowering cholesterol levels as a means of preventing coronary heart disease. For more information, see www.nhlbi.nih.gov/about/ncep/index.htm.

National Diabetes Education Program (NDEP): Federally sponsored initiative that involves public and private partners to improve the treatment and outcomes for people with diabetes, to promote early diagnosis, and ultimately to prevent the onset of diabetes. For more information, see www.cdc.gov/diabetes/projects/ndeps.htm.

Nephropathy: Kidney disease, a serious complication of diabetes.

Neuroendocrine: Pertaining to the interaction between the nervous and endocrine systems.

Neuropathy: Disease of the nervous system caused by damage to the nerves, a serious complication of diabetes.

Nutrients: Ingredients in food that provide nourishment. Proteins, carbohydrates, and fats are all essential nutrients that a healthy body needs to function.

Oral glucose tolerance test (OGTT): See *Glucose tolerance test.*

Osteoporosis: A disease characterized by a significant loss of bone density. Osteoporosis increases the risk of bone fractures or curvature of the spine.

Pancreas: The organ located behind the stomach that is responsible for producing insulin. Also produces and secretes other hormones and digestive chemicals called enzymes.

Periodontal disease: Disease of the gums; can be a complication of diabetes.

Peripheral vascular disease (PVD): Disease of the large blood vessels of the arms, legs, and feet caused by blocking of major blood vessels.

Pharmacotherapy: The treatment of disease with medicines.

Polycystic Ovary Syndrome (PCOS): A cluster of findings, including irregular menstrual periods and overproduction of the hormone androgen, with such signs as excess hair growth on the face, chest, and back. Other signs of PCOS are insulin resistance, obesity, acne, infertility, and cysts on the ovaries. Women with PCOS have a high risk for developing type 2 diabetes.

Prediabetes: A stage when glucose levels are higher than normal but not high enough to be considered diabetes. See also *Impaired fasting glucose* and *Impaired glucose tolerance.* Someone with prediabetes has a very high risk of developing diabetes and an increased risk of developing cardiovascular disease.

Preeclampsia: Condition characterized by high blood pressure that some women develop during the late stages of pregnancy. Preeclampsia is more common in women with diabetes.

Prevalence: The percentage of people in a given group who are reported to have a disease at a certain point in time.

Proliferative diabetic retinopathy (PDR): Growth of abnormal blood vessels and fibrous tissue from the inner retinal surface. A severe form of retinopathy.

Proteinuria: Too much protein in the urine; may be a sign of kidney damage.

Relative risk (RR): The ratio of the risk of death or disease in a specified group compared with a control population.

Renoprotective: Describes a factor that preserves kidney function or prevents kidney disease.

Retinopathy: A disease of the small blood vessels in the retina of the eye.

Self-efficacy: One's personal judgment of one's own ability to succeed in reaching a specific goal; belief in one's ability to maintain behavioral change in the face of situational challenges.

Self-management: A set of skilled behaviors that allow patients to manage their illnesses. For diabetes, this includes self-monitoring glucose management; taking medications for diabetes, blood pressure, and hyperlipidemia; adjusting diabetes medications as needed; and following dietary and activity guidelines and sick-day plans.

Sequelae: Results of a disease or injury or of complications. Sequelae of diabetes include its complications.

Social network: A set of social ties that connects an individual with others.

Social support: Emotional or task-oriented assistance provided by the community, family, friends, or significant others.

Socioeconomic status (SES): A descriptive term for a person's position in society, using criteria such as income, educational level attained, occupation, and value of dwelling place.

Stroke: Damage to the brain caused by blocked blood vessels in the brain. Depending on the part of the brain affected, stroke can cause loss of muscle function, mental function, vision, sensation, or speech. Diabetes increases the risk of stroke.

Sulfonylurea: A drug used to treat type 2 diabetes that increases insulin secretion and lowers the level of glucose (sugar) in the blood.

Thrombosis: The formation, development, or presence of a thrombus, or blood clot, in a blood vessel. Thrombosis can develop as a complication of atherosclerosis and is more common in people with diabetes.

Triglycerides: Type of blood fat.

United Kingdom Prospective Diabetes Study (UKPDS): Clinical study of newly diagnosed patients with type 2 diabetes. The UKPDS demonstrated that intensive glucose control prevents complications of diabetes.

Urinary incontinence: Uncontrollable loss of urine. There are two general types: urge incontinence, which is characterized by a sudden, uncontrollable urge to urinate; and stress incontinence, characterized by loss of urine after a physical activity such as sneezing, coughing, exercise, or laughing.

Urinary tract infections: Infections that occur when bacteria grow somewhere in the urinary tract (bladder or kidney).

Vaginitis: Any one of several types of inflammations of the vagina, caused by various organisms or by the low level of estrogen after menopause.

Vascular: Relating to the body's blood vessels (arteries, veins, capillaries). See *Cardiovascular disease.*

Vitreous hemorrhage: Bleeding into the clear jelly (gel) that fills the center of the eye.

Waist-to-hip ratio (WHR): A measure of central obesity, which is related to insulin resistance and diabetes risk. Formula: waist circumference divided by hip circumference.

References

CHAPTER 1: THE NEW EPIDEMIC

Beckles, G. L. A., and P. A. Thompson-Reid, eds. "Diabetes and Women's Health across the Life Stages: A Public Health Perspective." Atlanta, GA: U.S. Department of Health and Human Services, Centers for Disease Control and Prevention, Division of Diabetes Translation, 2001 (*www.cdc.gov/diabetes* or toll-free 1-877-CDC-DIAB).

Benjamin, S. M., et al. "Estimated Number of Adults with Pre-Diabetes in the United States in 2000: Opportunities for Prevention." *Diabetes Care,* 26(3) (March 2003): 645–649.

Department of Health and Human Services. "National Agenda for Public Health Action: The National Public Health Initiative on Diabetes and Women's Health." Atlanta, GA: Centers for Disease Control and Prevention, 2003.

Harris, M. I., et al. "Prevalence of Diabetes, Impaired Fasting Glucose, and Impaired Glucose Tolerance in U.S. Adults: The Third National Health and Nutrition Examination Survey, 1988–1994." *Diabetes Care,* 21(4) (1998): 518–524.

Ludwig, D. S., and C. B. Ebbeling. "Type 2 Diabetes Mellitus in Children: Primary Care and Public Health Considerations." *Journal of the American Medical Association,* 286 (2001): 1427–1430.

Morbidity and Mortality Weekly Report, "Socioeconomic Status of Women with Diabetes—United States, 2000." *Journal of the American Medical Association,* 287 (2002): 2542–2551.

Narayan, K. M., et al. "Lifetime Risk for Diabetes Mellitus in the United States." *Journal of the American Medical Association,* 290 (2003): 1884–1890.

"National Diabetes Statistics Fact Sheet: National Estimates and General Information on Diabetes in the United States." Bethesda, MD: U.S. Department of Health and Human Services, 2002.

CHAPTER 2: DIAGNOSIS

American Diabetes Association. "Diagnosis and Classification of Diabetes Mellitus." *Diabetes Care,* 27 (2004): S5–S10.

——. "Screening for Type 2 Diabetes (Position Statement)." *Diabetes Care,* 27 (2004): S11–S14.

——. Standards of Medical Care in Diabetes. *Diabetes Care,* 29(51) (2006): S4–S41.

Barr, R. G., et al. "Tests of Glycemia for the Diagnosis of Type 2 Diabetes Mellitus." *Annals of Internal Medicine,* 137(4) (2002): 263–272.

Copeland, K. C., et al. "Type 2 Diabetes in Children and Adolescents: Risk Factors, Diagnosis, and Treatment." *Clinical Diabetes,* 23 (2005): 181–185.

Davidson, M. B. "How Do We Diagnose Diabetes and Measure Blood Glucose Control?" *Diabetes Spectrum,* 14 (2001): 67–71.

Harris, R., et al. "Screening Adults for Type 2 Diabetes: A Review of the Evidence for the U.S. Preventive Services Task Force." *Annals of Internal Medicine,* 138(3) (2003): 215–229.

Meigs, J. B., et al. "The Natural History of Progression from Normal Glucose Tolerance to Type 2 Diabetes in the Baltimore Longitudinal Study of Aging." *Diabetes,* 52 (2003): 1475–1484.

National Diabetes Information Clearinghouse. "Insulin Resistance and Pre-Diabetes." NIH Publication No. 03–48393 (April 2003).

Sriram, U., and M. D. Rush. "Diabetes Overview." E-medicine consumer health website: www.emedicinehealth.com.

CHAPTER 3: PREVENTION

American Diabetes Association. "Evidence-Based Nutrition Principles and Recommendations for the Treatment and Prevention of Diabetes and Related Complications (Position Statement)." *Diabetes Care,* 25 (Supplement 1) (2002): S50–S60.

——. "Preventive Foot Care in Diabetes (Position Statement)." *Diabetes Care,* 27 (2004): S63–S64.

American Diabetes Association and the National Institute of Diabetes and Digestive and Kidney Disease. "Prevention or Delay of Type 2 Diabetes (Position Statement)." *Diabetes Care,* 26 (2003): S62–S69.

Barnard, R. J., et al. "Response of Noninsulin Dependent Diabetic Patients to an Intensive Program of Diet and Exercise." *Diabetes Care,* 5 (1982): 370.

———. "The Role of Diet and Exercise in the Management of Hyperinsulinemia and Associated Atherosclerosis Risk Factors." *American Journal of Cardiology,* 69 (1992): 330.

Diabetes Prevention Program. "DPP Lifestyle Materials and Optional Participant Handouts." Study documents website: www.bsc.gwu.edu/dpp/lifestyle/dpp_part.html.

Diabetes Prevention Program Research Group. "Description of Lifestyle Intervention." *Diabetes Care,* 25(12) (2002): 2165–2171.

———. "Reduction in the Incidence of Type 2 Diabetes with Lifestyle Intervention or Metformin." *New England Journal of Medicine,* 346 (2002): 393–403.

Franz, M. J. "So Many Nutrition Recommendations—Contradictory or Compatible?" *Diabetes Spectrum,* 16(1) (2003): 56–63.

Hu, F. B., et al. "Diet, Lifestyle and the Risk of Type 2 Diabetes in Women." *New England Journal of Medicine,* 345 (2001): 790–797. (For information about the Nurses' Health Study and other diabetes-related findings, see www.channing.harvard.edu/nhs.)

Mayfield, E. "A Consumer's Guide to Fats." *FDA Consumer* (January 1999).

National Diabetes Education Program. "Small Steps, Big Rewards: Your Game Plan for Preventing Type 2 Diabetes." NIH Publication No. 03–5334 (February 2003). Available online at ndep.nih.gov/materials/pubs/DPP/gameplan.pdf.

Ornish, D. M. *Dr. Dean Ornish's Program for Reversing Heart Disease.* New York: Random House, 1990.

Ornish, D. M., et al. "Can Lifestyle Changes Reverse Coronary Heart Disease?" *Lancet,* 336 (1990): 129.

Toobert, D. J., et al. "Biologic and Quality-of-Life Outcomes from the Mediterranean Lifestyle Program." *Diabetes Care,* 26 (2003): 2288–2293.

Torjesen, P. A., et al. "Lifestyle Changes May Reverse Development of the Insulin Resistance Syndrome." *Diabetes Care,* 20 (1) (1997): 26.

Tuomilehto, J., et al. "Prevention of Type 2 Diabetes Mellitus by Changes in Lifestyle among Subjects with Impaired Glucose Tolerance." Finnish Diabetes Prevention Study. *New England Journal of Medicine,* 344 (2001): 1343–1350.

Wing, R. R. "Very Low Calorie Diets in the Treatment of Type 2 Diabetes: Psychological and Physiological Effects." In T. A. Wadden and T. B.

Vanitallie, eds., *Treatment of the Seriously Obese Patient.* New York: Guilford, 1992.

CHAPTER 4: MEDICAL COMPLICATIONS

Adler, A. I., et al. "UKPDS 59: Hyperglycemia and Other Potentially Modifiable Risk Factors for Peripheral Vascular Disease in Type 2 Diabetes." *Diabetes Care,* 25 (2002): 894–899.

American Diabetes Association. "Hyperglycemic Crises in Patients with Diabetes Mellitus (Position Statement)." *Diabetes Care,* 26 (2003): S109–S117.

———. "Treatment of Hypertension in Adults with Diabetes (Position Statement)." *Diabetes Care,* 26 (2003): S80–S82.

Cho, E., et al. "A Prospective Study of Obesity and Risk of Coronary Heart Disease among Diabetic Women." *Diabetes Care,* 25(7) (2002): 1142–1148.

Colwell, J. A. "Aspirin Therapy in Diabetes (Technical Review)." *Diabetes Care,* 20 (1997): 1767–1771.

The Diabetes Control and Complications Trial Research Group. "The Effect of Intensive Treatment of Diabetes on the Development and Progression of Long-Term Complications in Insulin-Dependent Diabetes Mellitus." *New England Journal of Medicine,* 329(14) (1993): 977–986.

Diabetes Problems Prevention series, National Diabetes Information Clearinghouse. "Keep Your Diabetes under Control," "Keep Your Eyes Healthy," "Keep Your Feet and Skin Healthy," "Keep Your Heart and Blood Vessels Healthy," "Keep Your Kidneys Healthy," "Keep Your Nervous System Healthy," "Keep Your Teeth and Gums Healthy." Online at diabetes.niddk.nih.gov/dm/pubs/complications/index.htm.

Haffner, S. M. "Dyslipidemia Management in Adults with Diabetes." *Diabetes Care,* 27 (2004): S68–S71.

Haire-Joshu, D., et al. "Smoking and Diabetes (Technical Review)." *Diabetes Care,* 22 (1999): 1887–1898.

Henry, R. R. "Preventing Cardiovascular Complications of Type 2 Diabetes: Focus on Lipid Management." *Clinical Diabetes,* 19 (2001): 113–120.

Hu, F. B., et al. "The Impact of Diabetes Mellitus on Mortality from All Causes and Coronary Heart Disease in Women: Twenty Years of Follow-Up." *Archives of Internal Medicine,* 161 (2001): 1717–1723.

Koerbel, G., and M. Korytkowski. "Coronary Heart Disease in Women with Diabetes." *Diabetes Spectrum* (June 2003).

Nathan, D. M. "Long-Term Complications of Diabetes Mellitus." *New England Journal of Medicine,* 328 (1993): 1676–1685.

UK Prospective Diabetes Study Group. "Intensive Blood-Glucose Control with Sulphonylureas or Insulin Compared with Conventional Treatment and Risk of Complications in Patients with Type 2 Diabetes (UKPDS 33)." *Lancet,* 352 (1998): 837–853.

CHAPTER 5: REPRODUCTIVE HEALTH AND SEXUALITY

American Diabetes Association. "Gestational Diabetes Mellitus (Position Statement)." *Diabetes Care,* 27 (2004): S88–S90.

———. "Preconception Care of Women with Diabetes (Position Statement)." *Diabetes Care,* 27 (2004): S76–S78.

Dunne, F., et al. "Pregnancy in Women with Type 2 Diabetes: 12 Years Outcome Data 1990–2002." *Diabetes Medicine,* 20(9) (2003): 734–738.

Enzlin, P., et al. "Diabetes Mellitus and Female Sexuality: A Review of Twenty-five Years' Research." *Diabetic Medicine,* 15 (1998): 809–815.

Greene, M. F., and S. A. Eisenstat. "Diabetes in Pregnancy." Chapter 71 in *Primary Care of Women,* eds. K. J. Carlson and S. A. Eisenstat, 2nd ed. St. Louis: Mosby, 2002.

Hod, M., ed. *Textbook of Diabetes and Pregnancy.* London: Taylor and Francis, 2003.

Joslin Diabetes Center, Pregnancy Guideline Task Force. "Guideline for Detection and Management of Diabetes in Pregnancy." Updated September 14, 2005. Online at www.joslin.org/759_joslin_clinical_guidelines.asp.

Linne, Y. "Effects of Obesity on Women's Reproduction and Complications during Pregnancy." *Obesity Review,* 5(3) (2004): 137–143.

Lunt, H. "Women and Diabetes." *Diabetes Medicine,* 13 (1996): 1009–1016.

Nicodemus, K. K., and A. R. Folsom. "Type 1 and Type 2 Diabetes and Incident of Hip Fractures in Postmenopausal Women." *Diabetes Care,* 24 (2001): 1192–1197.

Sharpless, J. L. "Polycystic Ovary Syndrome and the Metabolic Syndrome. *Clinical Diabetes*, 21(4) (2003): 154–161.

Strotmeyer, E. S., et al. "Menstrual Cycle Differences between Women with Type 2 Diabetes and Women without Diabetes." *Diabetes Care*, 26 (2003): 1016–1021.

U.S. Food and Drug Administration. "Birth Control Guide." *FDA Consumer*. Updated December 2003.

Wu, P. "Thyroid Disease and Diabetes." *Clinical Diabetes*, 18(1) (2000): 38–41.

CHAPTER 6: PSYCHOSOCIAL IMPACT

Butler, D. "For Family Members Only." *Diabetes Self-Mangement* (2004). Online at http://www.diabetesselfmanagement.com/article.cfm?aid=1197.

Delahunty, L. M., et al. "Psychological and Behavioral Predictors of Weight Outcomes in the Diabetes Prevention Program." *Diabetes*, 51 (2002), supplement 2: A447.

Diabetes Prevention Program. "DPP Lifestyle Materials and Optional Participant Handouts." Handouts: "Overview of Strategies to Achieve Weight Loss," "The Slippery Slope of Lifestyle Change," "Problem Solving," "Talk Back to Negative Thoughts," "Take Charge of What's around You," "Make Social Cues Work *for* You," and "You Can Manage Stress." Study documents website: www.bsc.gwu.edu/dpp/lifestyle/dpp_part.html.

Holmes, D. M. "The Person and Diabetes in Psychosocial Context." *Diabetes Care*, 9(2) (1986): 194–206.

Howard, A. A., et al. "Effect of Alcohol Consumption on Diabetes Mellitus." *Annals of Internal Medicine*, 140(3) (2004): 211–219.

Jacobson, A. M. "The Psychological Care of Patients with Insulin-Dependent Diabetes Mellitus." *New England Journal of Medicine*, 334(19) (1996): 1249–1253.

Joslin Diabetes Center. "Diet Strategies for Women with Diabetes: Why Some Work and Why Some Don't." Online at www.joslin.org/managing _your_diabetes_694.asp.

Katon, W., et al. "Behavioral and Clinical Factors Associated with Depression among Individuals with Diabetes." *Diabetes Care*, 27 (2004): 914–920.

Lustman, P. J., and R. Anderson. "Depression in Adults with Diabetes." *Psychiatric Times*, 19(1) (January 2002).

Poirier-Solomon, L. "Eating Disorders and Diabetes—Brief Article." *Diabetes Forecast* (November 2001).

Rubin, R. R. "Dealing with 'Diabetes Overwhelmus.'" *Diabetes Self-Management* (2004). Online at www.diabetesselfmanagement.com/article.cfm?aid=434.

Rubin, R. R., and M. Peyrot. "Psychological Issues and Treatments for People with Diabetes." *Journal of Clinical Psychology,* 57(4) (2001): 457–478.

Surwit, R. S., et al. "Stress Management Improves Long-Term Glycemic Control in Type 2 Diabetes." *Diabetes Care,* 25 (2002): 30–34.

Wallhagen, M. I. "Social Support in Diabetes." *Diabetes Spectrum,* 12(4) (1999): 254–259.

Wurtman, R. J., and J. J. Wurtman. "Brain Serotonin, Carbohydrate-Craving, Obesity and Depression." *Obesity Research,* 3 (Supplement 4) (1995): 477S–480S.

CHAPTER 7: MANAGEMENT OF THE DISEASE

American Association of Clinical Endocrinologists. "Medical Guidelines for the Management of Diabetes Mellitus—2002 Update." *Endocrine Practice,* 8 (Supplement 1), January/February 2002.

American Diabetes Association. "Insulin Administration (Position Statement)." *Diabetes Care,* 24 (2001): 1984–1987.

———. "Influenza and Pneumococcal Immunization in Diabetes (Position Statement)." *Diabetes Care,* 27 (2004): S111–S113.

———. "Nutrition Principles and Recommendations in Diabetes (Position Statement)." *Diabetes Care,* 27 (2004): S36–S47.

———. "Physical Activity/Exercise and Diabetes (Position Statement)." *Diabetes Care,* 27 (2004): S58–S62.

———. "Tests of Glycemia in Diabetes (Position Statement)." *Diabetes Care,* 27 (2004): S91–S93.

———. "National Standards for Diabetes Self-Management Education (Standards and Review Criteria)." *Diabetes Care,* 28 (2005): S72–S79.

———. "Standards of Medical Care in Diabetes (Position Statement)." *Diabetes Care,* 28 (2005): S4–S36.

Centers for Disease Control and Prevention. *Take Charge of Your Diabetes,* 3rd ed. Atlanta: U.S. Department of Health and Human Services, 2003.

Chan, J. L., and M. J. Abrahamson. "Pharmacological Management of Type 2 Diabetes: Rationale for Rational Use of Insulin." *Mayo Clinic Proceedings,* 78(4) (2003): 411–413.

McCulloch, D. K. "Overview of Medical Care in Diabetes Mellitus" and "Nutritional Considerations in Diabetes Mellitus." UpToDate Online (online literature review service for physicians). Accessed 11/10/2004.

Nathan, D. M. "Initial Management of Glycemia in Type 2 Diabetes Mellitus." *New England Journal of Medicine,* 347(17) (2002): 1342–1349.

National Diabetes Information Clearinghouse. "Noninvasive Blood Glucose Monitors" (NIH Publication No. 04–4551, October 2003); "Medicines for People with Diabetes" (NIH Publication No. 03–4222, December 2002); "Devices for Taking Insulin" (NIH Publication No. 00–4643, February 2000).

Peragall-Dittko, V. "The Lowdown on Lancets and Lancing Devices." *Diabetes Self-Management,* 2004. Online at www.diabetesselfmanagement.com/article.cfm?aid=194.

———. "What's New in Blood Glucose Meters?" *Diabetes Self-Management,* 2004. Online at www.diabetesselfmanagement.com/article.cfm?aid=110.

Resource Guide 2005. "Oral Agents for Type 2" (RG8–9), "Insulin" (RG10–15), "Products for Testing Low Blood Glucose" (RG56–58), "Urine Testing" (RG59–63), "Insulin Delivery" (RG16–34), and "Blood Glucose Meters and Data Management Systems" (RG36–54). *Diabetes Forecast* (January 2005). Online at the American Diabetes Association's website: www.diabetes.org/diabetes-forecast/resource-guide.jsp.

CHAPTER 8: COMMON QUESTIONS AND RESOURCES

American Diabetes Association. "Smoking and Diabetes (Position Statement)." *Diabetes Care,* 27 (2004): S1–S2.

———. "Hypoglycemia and Employment/Licensure." *Diabetes Care,* 28 (2005): S61.

———. "Third-Party Reimbursement for Diabetes Care, Self-Management Education, and Supplies." *Diabetes Care,* 28 (2005): S62–S63.

———. "Your Guide to Eating Out." Online at www.diabetes.org/nutrition-and-recipes/nutrition/eatingoutguide.jsp. Accessed 10/25/05.

Chandran, M., and S. V. Edelman. "Have Insulin, Will Fly: Diabetes Management during Air Travel and Time Zone Adjustment Strategies." *Clinical Diabetes,* 21(2) (2003): 82–84.

Cox, D. J., et. al. "Diabetes and Driving Mishaps: Frequency and Correlations from a Multinational Survey." *Diabetes Care,* 26(8) (2003): 2464–2465.

Diabetes Prevention Program. "DPP Lifestyle Materials and Optional Participant Handouts." "Session 10: Four Keys to Healthy Eating Out." Study documents website: www.bsc.gwu.edu/dpp/lifestyle/dpp_part.html.

Fabricatore, A. N., and T. A. Wadden. "Treatment of Obesity: An Overview." *Clinical Diabetes,* 21 (2003): 61–72.

Harris, M. I. "Health Insurance and Diabetes." Chapter 29 in *Diabetes in America,* 2nd ed. National Diabetes Data Group, National Institutes of Health, National Institute of Diabetes and Digestive and Kidney Diseases, NIH Publication No. 95–1468 (1995).

Journal of the American Medical Association Patient Page. "Safe Driving for People with Diabetes." *Journal of the American Medical Association,* 282(8) (1999): 806.

O'Connell, T. L. "An Overview of Obesity and Weight Loss Surgery." *Clinical Diabetes,* 22 (2004): 115–120.

Tibbs, T. L., and D. Haire-Joshu. "Avoiding High-Risk Behaviors: Smoking Prevention and Cessation in Diabetes Care." *Diabetes Spectrum,* 15 (2002): 164–169.

Weight-Control Information Network, National Institute of Diabetes and Digestive and Kidney Diseases. "Prescription Medications for the Treatment of Obesity." NIH Publication No. 04–4191 (November 2004). Online at win.niddk.nih.gov/publications/prescription.htm.

Yeh, G. Y., et al. "Systematic Review of Herbs and Dietary Supplements for Glycemic Control in Diabetes." *Diabetes Care,* 26(4) (2003): 1277–1294.

Acknowledgments

We would like to thank the two anonymous reviewers for Harvard University Press for providing an excellent technical review of an early draft of the manuscript. Their comments were immensely helpful as we made our revisions. We would also like to acknowledge the professionalism and persistence of those at Harvard University Press who have worked so hard on *Every Woman's Guide to Diabetes*: Ann Downer-Hazell, our sponsoring editor, whose sound advice has informed every page of this book; Bethany Withers and Alissa Anderson, who answered our questions about manuscript preparation and helped organize the artwork and tables; Christine Thorsteinsson, who copyedited the manuscript and shepherded it through production; Susan Thomas, who prepared the index; Deborah Hodgdon, who devised a beautiful design inside and out; and Jerry Kaplan, who coordinated the book's production. William P. Sisler and Michael G. Fisher provided crucial support for the project from its earliest stages. Medical illustrator Arleen Frasca drew the original line illustrations, accommodating our requests for changes with grace and good will. Their invaluable contributions have made this a better book.

Finally, we'd like to thank our colleagues and our patients, who inform our practice every day.

Index

Note: Page numbers followed by t refer to tables.

Acanthosis nigricans, 23
Acarbose, 194t
ACE inhibitors. *See* Angiotensin-converting enzyme (ACE) inhibitors
Acesultame-potassium, 68t
Adolescents, diabetes in, 113–114
African Americans, diabetes in, 2, 11, 13, 175
Airline travel, 232–236
Alaska natives, diabetes in, 11, 12
Alcohol use, 165–167, 166t
Alpha blockers, 84t
Alpha-glucosidase inhibitors, 192t, 194t
Alprazolam, 163t
Alternative medicine treatments, 248–250, 274–275
American Association of Diabetes Educators, 254
American Diabetes Association, 254
American Dietetic Association, 254
American Heart Association, 255
American Indians, diabetes in, 2, 11, 12, 14
American Obesity Association, 255
Americans with Disabilities Act, 238–239
Amitriptyline, 163t
Amputation, 16, 78, 85, 95, 97, 103
Angiotensin-converting enzyme (ACE) inhibitors, 83, 84t, 85, 101, 129, 223t, 277
Angiotensin II receptor blocker (ARB), 83, 84t, 85, 101
Annual examination, 222, 223t–224t
Anorexia nervosa, 168
Antianxiety agents, 163t
Antidepressants, 162, 163t
Antidiarrheal medications, 273
Antihypertensives, 83–85, 84t
Anxiety, 159–161

ARB. *See* Angiotensin II receptor blocker (ARB)
Arteriosclerosis, 85, 86, 90, 94
Artificial sweeteners, 68t
Asian Americans, diabetes in, 2, 13–14
Aspartame, 68t
Aspirin, 91, 273
Atherosclerosis, 46, 93, 277, 278
Autonomic neuropathy, 102, 103, 278

Bariatric surgery, 243–244
Basal insulin, 182t, 195, 203, 236, 278
Benzodiazepines, 163t
Beta blockers, 84t, 163t
Beta cells, 4, 6–8, 9, 24, 38, 278
Biguanides, 192t, 194t
Bile acid sequestrants, 88
Binge eating disorder, 168–170
Birth weight, 23
Blindness, 15–16, 98–100
Blood glucose. *See* Glucose, blood
Blood pressure: control of, 82–85; goals for, 276; high, 21, 82–85, 84t
Blood sugar log, 184–188, 221, 223t, 227, 267
Blurred vision, 100
Body mass index (BMI), 41, 255, 260–261
Bolus insulin, 195, 203, 204, 278
Bone density scan, 147
Breastfeeding, 139–140
Bulimia, 168
Bupropion, 163t
Burn-out, 154–155
Buspirone, 163t
Byetta, 193

Calcium, 66, 209
Calcium channel blockers, 84t

Calories, 49–57, 61–64, 165–166, 206, 217t

Carbohydrates, 204, 208–210; counting of, 204–205, 212–215, 262–263; counts for common foods, 262–263; glycemic index of, 213–214

Cardiovascular disease. *See* Heart disease; Peripheral vascular disease; Stroke

Carpal tunnel syndrome, 102

Cataracts, 98

Centers for Disease Control and Prevention, 255

Central adiposity, 47, 278, 287

Cerebrovascular disease, 278

Cervical cap, 125

Cheating, 154

Children: diabetes in, 3–4, 23–24, 113–114, 130; diabetes prevention for, 72–73

Cholesterol, 21–22, 58, 85–89, 87t; goals for, 87t, 223t, 276; HDL, 85–87, 281; LDL, 85–87, 283; lowering by medication, 88. *See also* Triglycerides

Cholesterol absorption inhibitors, 88

Cigarette smoking, cessation of, 89, 240–242

Citalopram, 163t

Clinical trials, 42–45, 251–252

Clomipramine, 163t

Clonazepam, 163t

Cold medicines, 229, 273

Coma, 108

Combined alpha and beta blockers, 84t

Complementary (alternative medicine) treatments, 248–250, 274–275

Complications, 14–16, 74–111; blood pressure control for, 82–85; cardiovascular, 15, 75–76, 77, 78, 79, 90–97; cholesterol profile in, 85–89; emergency, 78; glucose control for, 79–82; macrovascular, 75–76, 77, 78, 79, 90–97; management of, 220–224, 223t–224t; metabolic, 106–110; microvascular, 77, 78, 79, 97–106; nervous system, 77, 78, 101–105, 104t; oc-

ular, 15–16, 98–100; periodontal, 16, 77, 78, 105–106; during pregnancy, 78, 127, 131; prevention of, 79–89; renal, 16, 77, 100–101; skin, 77, 78, 106, 107t

Condom, 121t, 124

Congenital malformations, 78, 127–128, 135, 280

Contraception, 120–126, 121t; barrier, 121t, 124–125; emergency, 126; injection for, 121t, 123–124; IUD, 121t, 125; oral, 121t, 122–123; patch for, 123; ring for, 123; sponge for, 125

Coronary artery disease, 3, 15, 85, 90–97; cholesterol levels in, 85–89; death from, 92–93; hormone replacement therapy and, 142; prevention of, 75–76

Coronary heart disease. See Heart disease

Cough medicines, 229, 273

Culture, 174–177, 247–248

Delivery, 138–139

Dental disease, 16, 77, 78, 105–106

Depo-Provera, 121t, 123–124

Depression, 91, 151, 161–164, 163t

Desipramine, 163t

Desserts, 67

Diabetes Control and Complications Trial, 81

Diabetes mellitus: adolescents, 113–114; children, 23–24, 72–73, 130; correcting misconceptions, 15; epidemic of, 10–14; epidemiology of, 1, 3; etiology, 5; natural history, 7; type 1, 5, 6, 9; type 2, 5, 6–8, 9. *See also* Medications

Diabetes nurse educator, 34

Diabetes Prevention Program, 38–40, 43–44, 47, 172–173, 256

Diabetes targets, 276

Diabetic ketoacidosis, 20–21, 106–107

Diagnosis, 18–36; in children, 23–24; reactions to, 30–31, 151–153; risk factors in, 21–23; symptoms in, 19–21; testing in, 24–30, 29t

Dialysis, 101

Diaphragm, 121t, 124–125

Diet, 3–4, 204–212; balanced, 55–57, 204; for complication prevention, 89; food portions in, 207; food pyramids for, 56, 57; grocery list for, 265; medical nutrition therapy for, 204–206; mood and, 171–174; nutrients in, 206–212; during pregnancy, 137–138; for weight loss, 50–51, 52t. *See also* Carbohydrates; Fats; Weight loss
Dietitian, 34–35
Disposing of syringes, 270
Diuretics, 84t
Driving, 236–237
Drugs. *See* Medications
Dyslipidemia, 85–89
Dysthymic disorder, 162

Eating disorders, 167–174; emotion and, 54–55, 171–174; self-assessment for, 170–171
Eating out, 239–240
Eclampsia. *See* Preeclampsia/eclampsia
Edema, macular, 98
Emergencies, 231
Emergency contraception, 126
Emotion. *See* Psychosocial factors
Employment, 237–239
Endometrial cancer, 120, 122, 142, 147
Escitalopram, 163t
Estrogen, glucose control and, 115, 116
Ethnicity, diabetes and, 2, 11–14, 175
Etiology, of diabetes, 5
Exchange lists, 212
Exenatide, 191
Exercise: heart rate for, 218, 219; during pregnancy, 131–132; types of, 70t; for weight loss, 8, 38–40, 55, 68–72, 70t, 216–217, 217t
Eye disease, 15–16, 98–100

Family practitioner, 31, 33
Family support, 176–177
Fasting blood glucose 10; fasting plasma glucose test, 20, 25–27; for gestational diabetes, 136
Fats, 206–208; food labeling for, 60–64;

recipe modification for, 65–66; restriction of, 51–52, 58–59, 66–68; types of, 58–59
Fenfluramine, 243
Fetal malformations, 78, 127–128, 135, 280
Fiber, 210–212
Fibrates, 88
Fingerstick, 186–187
Finnish Diabetes Prevention study, 43
Flu, 232; flu shot, 232
Fluoxetine, 163t
Fluvoxamine, 163t
Folic acid, 129
Food. *See* Diet; Weight loss
Food diary, 59–60
Food labels, 60–64
Food pyramid: new Willett, 57; original, 56
Foot disorders, 94–97, 95t, 103–104; prevention of, 104–105, 104t
Free fatty acids, 46–47

Gastric bypass, 243–244
Gestational diabetes mellitus (GDM), 2, 8–9, 134–137; screening for, 27, 135, 136, 136t; type 2 diabetes and, 137
Glaucoma, 98
Glimepiride, 194t
Glipizide, 194t
Glossary, 277–287
Glucose, blood, 180–190; continuous monitoring of, 188; control of, 79–82; elevation of, 4, 7, 106–108; fingerstick for, 186–187; goals for, 80, 183–184, 276; during illness, 229; insulin production and, 4; log for, 185, 187–188; low, 108–110, 132, 148; menstrual cycle and, 114–119; meter for, 184–188, 266–268; monitoring of, 180–183, 182t; normalization of, 190–193, 192t; schedule, 182t; stress effects on, 156, 229; testing sites for, 189; test strips for, 185–186. *See also* Insulin; Weight loss
Glucose tolerance test, 10, 20, 27; for gestational diabetes, 136, 136t
Glyburide, 194t

Glycemic index, 213–214
Glycohemoglobin (HgbA$_{1c}$) test, 28–30, 29t, 182–183; during pregnancy, 128; target for, 80, 81
Graves' disease, 145–146
Grocery list, 264–265
Gum disease, 16, 77, 78, 105–106

Hawaiian Americans, diabetes in, 13–14
HDL cholesterol. See Cholesterol, HDL
Health insurance, 3, 250–251
Healthy snacks, 66, 67
Heart attack, 3, 90, 93
Heart disease, 3, 15, 90–97; cholesterol levels and, 85–89; death from, 92–93; hormone replacement therapy and, 142; prevention of, 75–76
Heart rate, for exercise, 218, 219
Hemoglobin A$_{1c}$ (HgbA$_{1c}$), 28–30, 29t, 182–183; during pregnancy, 128; target for, 29, 80, 81
Herbal treatments, 248–250, 274–275
High blood pressure. See Hypertension
Hispanic Americans, diabetes in, 11, 13
HMG CoA reductase inhibitors, 88
Hormone replacement therapy, 91, 141–142
Hyperglycemia, 4, 7, 106–110
Hyperinsulinemia, 282. See also Insulin resistance
Hyperosmolar hyperglycemic, nonketotic coma, 108, 109
Hypertension, 82–85; definition of, 83; treatment of, 83–85, 84t
Hyperthyroidism, 145–146
Hypoglycemia, 108–110; during pregnancy, 132; sexual activity and, 148
Hypothyroidism, 145–146

Illness, management of, 228–232
Impaired glucose tolerance (IGT), 27, 28, 282
Incontinence, 143, 145
Infection: skin, 106; urinary tract, 141, 143; yeast, 141, 142–143
Infertility, 130

Injection contraception, 123–124
Insulin, 4, 191, 193–203, 269; basal, 195; bolus, 195; daily schedule and, 35; errors in, 201; during illness, 229; inhalation of, 202–203, 271; injection methods for, 198–202; intentional omission of, 169, 170; jet injectors for, 202, 271; mixing, 269; patches for, 203; pens for, 202, 271; during pregnancy, 129–130, 133, 134; problems with, 198t, 201, 202; pump for, 203, 271, 272; for travel, 235–236; types of, 196t–197t. See also Basal insulin; Bolus insulin
Insulin resistance, 6, 7, 8; depression and, 164; obesity and, 46
Intensive diabetes control, 76
Intensive glucose control, 79–82, 283; in pregnancy, 127–128
Internet resources, 253–256
Internist, 31, 33
Intrauterine device, 121t, 125
Ischemic heart disease. See Heart disease

Ketoacidosis, 20–21, 106–107; during pregnancy, 133
Ketone testing, 107–108, 189–190
Kidney disease, 16, 77, 100–101

Labor, 138–139
Laser therapy, in retinopathy, 100
Latino Americans, diabetes in, 11, 13
LDL cholesterol. See Cholesterol, LDL
Libido, 148
Lifestyle modifications: clinical trials of, 42–45; Diabetes Prevention Program study of, 38–39, 43–44, 52–53; Finnish Diabetes Prevention study of, 43; for hypertension, 83; motivation for, 47–49; Nurses' Health study of, 44–45; typical day and, 32t–33t. See also Diet; Weight loss
Lipids. See Cholesterol
Lipoproteins: high-density, 85, 87t; low-density, 85, 87t
Lorazepam, 163t
Low blood sugar. See Hypoglycemia

Macrosomia, 133–134
Macrovascular disease, 78, 90–97, 283–284
Macular edema, 98
Medical care: annual, 222, 223t–224t; culture and, 247–248; emergency, 231; guidelines, 223; for minor illness, 228–232; for nutrition, 204–206; team for, 226
Medical identification, 233, 234
Medications: abuse of, 166; antianxiety, 163t; antidepressant, 162, 163t; antidiarrheal, 273; antihypertensive, 83–85, 84t; anti-inflammatory, 273; during breastfeeding, 139; cholesterol-lowering, 88; common problems with, 198t; for diabetes prevention, 45–46; oral antidiabetic, 191–193, 192t, 194t; during pregnancy, 129; for weight loss, 45–46, 216. See also Insulin
Meglitinides, 192t, 194t
Menopause, 140–142, 245
Menstrual cycle, 115, 116–117; glucose control and, 114–119; irregularities in, 118–119; normal, 115; premenstrual syndrome and, 118
Metabolic complications, 106–110
Metabolic syndrome, 10, 47
Metformin, 191, 194t
Microalbuminuria, 101
Microvascular disease, 78, 97–101, 284
Miglitol, 194t
Mirtazapine, 163t
Miscarriage, 130
Misconceptions, 15
Monoamine oxidase inhibitors, 163t
Myocardial infarction, 3, 90, 93

Nateglinide, 194t
National Diabetes Information Clearinghouse, 256
National Women's Health Information Center, 256
Native Americans, 11, 12, 13, 135, 247
Nefazodone, 163t

Nephropathy, 16, 77, 100–101
Nerve problems. See Neuropathy
Neuropathy, 16, 77, 78, 101–105, 104t
Niacin, 88
Nonsteroidal anti-inflammatory drugs (NSAIDs), 273
Nurse educator, 34
Nurses' Health Study, 44–45
Nursing, 139–140
Nutrition, 89, 204–212. See also Diet; Weight loss
Nutritional guidelines, 206
Nutrition Facts label, 60–64

Obesity, 10–11, 21; employment and, 239; endometrial cancer and, 147; extreme, 242–244; free fatty acids and, 46–47; insulin resistance and, 46; pregnancy and, 134; psychosocial effects of, 164–165; type of, 47. See also Central adiposity; Weight loss
Older women, 246–247
Oral antidiabetic agents, 191–193, 192t, 194t
Oral contraceptives, 120, 121t, 122–123
Oral glucose tolerance test, 10, 20, 27; for gestational diabetes, 136, 136t
Organizing supplies, 226
Orlistat, 243
Osteoporosis, 146

Pacific Islanders, diabetes in, 2, 13–14
Pancreas, 4
Panic disorder, 160
Paroxetine, 163t
Periodontal disease, 16, 77, 78, 105–106
Peripheral nerve disorders, 101–105, 104t
Peripheral vascular disease, 90, 94–97, 95t
Phenelzine, 163t
Physical activity: during pregnancy, 131–132; for weight loss, 8, 38–40, 55, 68–72, 70t, 216–220, 217t
Physician, 31, 33
Pima Indians, diabetes in, 12

Pioglitazone, 194t
Plasma glucose test: fasting, 10, 20, 25–27, 136; random, 25
Pneumonia vaccine, 224t, 232, 276
Polycystic ovary syndrome (PCOS), 119–120, 130, 244
Portion size, 64, 65t, 66, 207, 212, 240
Post-coital contraception, 126
Pramlintide, 191
Prediabetes, 7, 9–10, 22; diagnosis of, 10, 25–27; risk for, 40–41
Preeclampsia/eclampsia, 78, 127, 133, 280, 285
Pregnancy, 112, 244–245; breastfeeding (nursing), 123, 139–140; complications during, 127, 128, 131; diabetes screening in, 135, 136, 136t; fetal complications, 127; gestational diabetes and, 2, 8–9, 27, 134–137, 136t; glucose control during, 128–130, 133–134; hemoglobin A$_{1c}$ during, 128; hypoglycemia during, 132; insulin during, 129–130, 133, 134; labor and delivery, 138–139; maternal complications, 127; medications during, 129; nutrition during, 137–138; physical activity during, 131–132; physical examination in, 129; planning for, 126–130; safe medications, 129; type 1 diabetes and, 132–134, 133t; type 2 diabetes and, 134
Premature labor, 78, 127, 133
Premenstrual syndrome, 118, 160
Prevention, 37–73; in children, 72–73; clinical trials of, 42–45; of complications, 79–89; Diabetes Prevention Program study of, 43–44, 47; exercise in, 39–40; Finnish Diabetes Prevention study of, 43; medications for, 45–46; motivation for, 47–49; Nurses' Health Study of, 44–45; weight loss in, 39, 46–47, 49–51, 52t
Primary care physician, 31, 33
Progesterone, glucose control and, 115, 116
Proliferative diabetic retinopathy, 98
Propranolol, 163t

Protein, dietary, 208
Proteinuria, 285. See also Kidney disease
Psychosocial factors, 150–177; alcohol abuse and, 165–167; culture and, 174–177; daily adjustments and, 153–156; depression and, 161–164, 163t; diagnosis and, 30–31, 151–153; drug abuse and, 165–167; eating disorders and, 54–55, 167–174; family support and, 176–177; obesity and, 164–165; positive perspective on, 177; self-assessment for, 155–156, 170–171; stress and, 156–159; worry and, 159–161
Pulse, for exercise, 219
Purging. See Eating disorders

Racism, 175
Random plasma glucose test, 25
Relaxation therapy, 157–158
Repaglinide, 194t
Resources, 71–72, 253–256
Restaurants, 239–240
Retina, 99
Retinopathy, 15–16, 98–100
Risk, 41–42
Risk factors, 2, 21–23; for prediabetes, 40–41
Rosiglitazone, 194t

Saccharin, 68t
Safety: for driving, 236–237; for exercise, 220
Saturated fats, 58, 59
Screening, 22–23; for children, 23–24
Self-management, 179–180
Serotonin reuptake inhibitors, 163t
Sertraline, 163t
Setting goals, 54
Sexism, 175, 176
Sexual function, 147–148
Sibutramine, 243
Sick-day plan, 228–232
Skin disorders, 95, 95t, 104–105, 104t, 106, 107t
Smoking cessation, 89
Snacks, 66, 67

Social anxiety disorder, 160
Specialists, 35–36
Sponge, contraceptive, 125
Statins, 88
Sterilization, 126
Stress, 156–159, 229; management of, 157–158
Stroke, 15, 90, 93–94
Substance abuse, 165–167
Sucralose, 68t
Sugar. *See* Glucose
Sugars, commercial, 68t, 209–210
Sulfonylureas, 191, 192t, 194t
Superwoman complex, 174
Supplies, 226–227; meter, 184–186, 266–268; payment for, 250–251; pump, 271–272; syringe container, 270; test strip, 185–186; for travel, 232–236
Sweeteners, 68t, 209–210
Symptoms, 19–21
Syringes, disposing of, 270

Target heart rate, 218
Test strips, 185–186
Thiazolidinediones, 192t, 194t
Thyroid disease, 145–146
Time management, 227–228
Trans fatty acids, 58, 59
Transient ischemic attack, 94
Travel, 232–236
Tricyclic antidepressants, 163t
Triglycerides, 22, 85–89, 87t, 282
Tubal ligation, 121t, 126
Tylenol, 273
Type 1 diabetes. *See* Diabetes mellitus, type 1
Type 2 diabetes. *See* Diabetes mellitus, type 2

Ulcers, foot, 95, 95t, 104–105, 104t
United Kingdom Prospective Diabetes Study, 82

Unsaturated fats, 58, 59
Urinary incontinence, 143, 145
Urinary ketones, 107–108, 189–190
Urinary tract, 144; infection of, 141, 143
Uterine cancer. *See* Endometrial cancer

Vagina: dryness of, 147–148; infection of, 141, 142–143
Vaginal contraceptive ring, 123
Vaginitis, 143
Vasectomy, 126
Vasodilators, 84t
Venlafaxine, 163t
Vision loss, 15–16
Vitrectomy, 100

Websites, 253–256
Weight-Control Information Network, 256
Weight loss, 46–47, 164–165, 215–220; balanced diet and, 55–57; clinical trials of, 42–45; counseling for, 52–53; Diabetes Prevention Program study of, 38–40, 43–44, 52–53, 172–173; diets for, 49–51, 52t, 55–57; emotion and, 54–55, 171–174; in extreme obesity, 242–244; fat restriction for, 51–52, 58–59; food diary for, 59–60; food labels for, 60–64; goals for, 39, 54, 205, 206, 215; insulin omission and, 169, 170; medications for, 45–46, 216; motivation for, 47–49; options, 51; physical activity for, 38, 55, 68–72, 70t, 216–220, 217t; portion sizes for, 65t; problem solving for, 171–173; recipe modification for, 65–66, 65t; successful, 51–53; surgery for, 243–244
Worry, 159–161

Yeast infection, 141, 142–143